Biomedical
Ethics OPPOSING VIEWPOINTS®

Other Books of Related Interest in the Opposing
Viewpoints Series:

Abortion
AIDS
American Values
Animal Rights
Constructing a Life Philosophy
Death and Dying
The Elderly
Euthanasia
Genetic Engineering
Global Resources
The Health Crisis
Science and Religion

Biomedical Ethics
OPPOSING VIEWPOINTS®

David Bender & Bruno Leone, *Series Editors*

Terry O'Neill, *Book Editor*

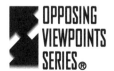

OPPOSING
VIEWPOINTS
SERIES®

Greenhaven Press, Inc.   PO Box 289009   San Diego, CA 92198-9009

Library of Congress Cataloging-in-Publication Data

Biomedical ethics : opposing viewpoints / Terry O'Neill, book
    editor.
        p.   cm. — (Opposing viewpoints series)
    Includes bibliographical references and index.
    Summary: Presents opposing viewpoints on biomedical
ethics issues such as genetic engineering, organ transplants,
medical use of fetal tissue, and reproductive technology.
    ISBN 1-56510-062-X (lib. : acid-free paper) — ISBN 1-56510-
061-1 (pbk. : acid-free paper)
    1. Medical ethics. 2. Bioethics. [1. Medical ethics. 2.
Bioethics.] I. O'Neill, Terry, 1944–   . II. Series: Opposing
viewpoints series (Unnumbered)
R724.B492 1994
174'.2—dc20   93-7260
                                                              CIP
                                                               AC

"Congress shall make no law . . . abridging the freedom of speech, or of the press."

First Amendment to the U.S. Constitution

The basic foundation of our democracy is the first amendment guarantee of freedom of expression. The Opposing Viewpoints Series is dedicated to the concept of this basic freedom and the idea that it is more important to practice it than to enshrine it.

Contents

Why Consider Opposing Viewpoints?

"The only way in which a human being can make some approach to knowing the whole of a subject is by hearing what can be said about it by persons of every variety of opinion and studying all modes in which it can be looked at by every character of mind. No wise man ever acquired his wisdom in any mode but this."

John Stuart Mill

In our media-intensive culture it is not difficult to find differing opinions. Thousands of newspapers and magazines and dozens of radio and television talk shows resound with differing points of view. The difficulty lies in deciding which opinion to agree with and which "experts" seem the most credible. The more inundated we become with differing opinions and claims, the more essential it is to hone critical reading and thinking skills to evaluate these ideas. Opposing Viewpoints books address this problem directly by presenting stimulating debates that can be used to enhance and teach these skills. The varied opinions contained in each book examine many different aspects of a single issue. While examining these conveniently edited opposing views, readers can develop critical thinking skills such as the ability to compare and contrast authors' credibility, facts, argumentation styles, use of persuasive techniques, and other stylistic tools. In short, the Opposing Viewpoints Series is an ideal way to attain the higher-level thinking and reading skills so essential in a culture of diverse and contradictory opinions.

In addition to providing a tool for critical thinking, Opposing Viewpoints books challenge readers to question their own strongly held opinions and assumptions. Most people form their opinions on the basis of upbringing, peer pressure, and personal, cultural, or professional bias. By reading carefully balanced opposing views, readers must directly confront new ideas as well as the opinions of those with whom they disagree. This is not to simplistically argue that everyone who reads opposing views will—or should—change his or her opinion. Instead, the series enhances readers' depth of understanding of their own views by encouraging confrontation with opposing ideas. Careful examination of others' views can lead to the readers' understanding of the logical inconsistencies in their own opinions, perspective on why they hold an opinion, and the consideration of the possibility that their opinion requires further evaluation.

Evaluating Other Opinions

To ensure that this type of examination occurs, Opposing Viewpoints books present all types of opinions. Prominent spokespeople on different sides of each issue as well as well-known professionals from many disciplines challenge the reader. An additional goal of the series is to provide a forum for other, less known, or even unpopular viewpoints. The opinion of an ordinary person who has had to make the decision to cut off life support from a terminally ill relative, for example, may be just as valuable and provide just as much insight as a medical ethicist's professional opinion. The editors have two additional purposes in including these less known views. One, the editors encourage readers to respect others' opinions—even when not enhanced by professional credibility. It is only by reading or listening to and objectively evaluating others' ideas that one can determine whether they are worthy of consideration. Two, the inclusion of such viewpoints encourages the important critical thinking skill of objectively evaluating an author's credentials and bias. This evaluation will illuminate an author's reasons for taking a particular stance on an issue and will aid in readers' evaluation of the author's ideas.

As series editors of the Opposing Viewpoints Series, it is our hope that these books will give readers a deeper understanding of the issues debated and an appreciation of the complexity of even seemingly simple issues when good and honest people disagree. This awareness is particularly important in a democratic society such as ours in which people enter into public debate to determine the common good. Those with whom one disagrees should not be regarded as enemies but rather as people whose views deserve careful examination and may shed light on one's own.

Thomas Jefferson once said that "difference of opinion leads to inquiry, and inquiry to truth." Jefferson, a broadly educated man, argued that "if a nation expects to be ignorant and free . . . it expects what never was and never will be." As individuals and as a nation, it is imperative that we consider the opinions of others and examine them with skill and discernment. The Opposing Viewpoints Series is intended to help readers achieve this goal.

David L. Bender & Bruno Leone,
Series Editors

Introduction

"From the nineteenth-century view of science as a god, the twentieth century has begun to see it as a devil. It behooves us now to understand that science is neither one nor the other."

Agnes Meyer, Education for a New Morality, *1957*

The insatiable thirst for knowledge is a uniquely human trait. But that thirst is not without peril. The biblical story of the Garden of Eden illustrates the view many people hold—that in the search for knowledge it is possible to go too far, in a sense to seek to be God. Today those involved in biomedical technology are often criticized for this tendency.

In the twentieth century, science has advanced far beyond what our ancestors dared imagine. Today scientists can cure diseases that used to wipe out entire civilizations. They can enable an infertile couple to bear children. They can prolong the life of the terminally ill and replace the damaged organs of those suffering from kidney or heart disease. They can diagnose and sometimes prevent mental and physical disease before a child is born.

But the line between what can be done and what should be done is sometimes very thin. For example, science makes it possible for a postmenopausal woman to bear a child. But just because it can be done, should it be done? Critics point out the stresses the older mother's body would undergo and the likelihood that she would die while her child was still young. Science makes it possible to determine the sex of a child within a few days after it has been conceived. But critics fear this knowledge will be used to abort healthy children merely because of their gender. Science may soon make it possible to remove a "violence gene" from the genetic makeup of a fetus, or to add a "tall gene," a "beauty gene," or a "smart gene." But, critics ask, is it right to tamper with human life in this way? Critics fear that just as generations of special breeding have made some classes of dogs highstrung to the point where they are no longer good family pets, so could genetic engineering of humans lead to unforeseen results. Placing in the hands of a few scientists the awesome power of human destiny conjures up images of

Frankenstein or Jurassic Park. Many wonder if such power would defy and disrupt some ultimate, unknowable plan for the universe.

But those who support the advances of biomedical technology point out that the scientific community is not made up of mad scientists run amok. In fact, they say, scientists give grave thought to the consequences of the tasks they undertake, and the results, overall, benefit humanity. While science perhaps should not do *everything* it can do, they believe it would be a tragedy not to continue seeking new knowledge. Many scientists today would echo the words Francis P. Cobbe wrote in 1887: "Then the sorcerer Science entered, and where e'er he waved his wand,/ Fresh wonders and fresh mysteries rose on every hand."

This book replaces Greenhaven Press's 1987 title of the same name with all new viewpoints. The authors in this book consider many facets of the complex world of biomedical ethics today. The issues include What Ethics Should Guide Biomedical Research? What Ethics Should Guide Organ Transplants? What Ethics Should Guide Fetal Tissue Research? Are Reproductive Technologies Ethical? Should Animals Be Used in Research? What Ethics Should Guide Genetic Research?

What Ethics Should Guide Biomedical Research?

Biomedical Ethics

Chapter Preface

Recent great advances in science have led to a host of ethical questions unimaginable in times past. These include questions about ownership of biomedical products.

Those who invent new machines or parts for them or other nonliving products have traditionally been able to patent and profit from them. The ownership of new developments in living "products" has been more controversial. Many people are not opposed to patenting a new tomato that resists rot or a new breed of pig that produces leaner meat. But some become uneasy when it comes to patenting a new mouse developed through genetic manipulation specifically to spontaneously contract breast cancer. Even more sensitive is the idea of patenting human cells or products made from them.

One of the first such cases made the news in 1984. A patient's abnormal spleen cells, unbeknownst to him, were used to develop a human cell line for medical research. The cell line was patented by the developer, the man's doctor, and has subsequently earned a great deal of money for the developer but none for the patient. This case raised a plethora of ethical questions. Among them: Should a doctor be able to use a patient's cells for research without the patient's explicit consent? Should the doctor profit, and not the patient from whose body the cells were taken? Should human by-products be patentable in any event?

Many think the human body should be sacrosanct and that the work of scientists should be divorced from the profit motive. Others say human by-products are really no different from the by-products of animal or plant research and that profit is the motive that enables scientific research to be supported at all. The government cannot support all research that can be done, they note, and private companies will not support research for which there is no hope of profit.

The authors of the following viewpoints discuss some of the ethical questions relating to the patenting of biomedical products and to the use of human subjects in research, another highly sensitive area in biomedical ethics.

"The tremendous cost of developing a new biotechnology product . . . [makes] clear and meaningful patent protection . . . essential."

Biological Patents Promote Progress

Lisa J. Raines

Few people question the right of a scientist to patent and subsequently profit from his or her invention of a new kind of sticky tape, a new computer chip, or a new auto manifold. The patenting of living things, however, is more controversial. With advances in genetic research, some scientists are now trying to obtain patents on new cells they have developed by altering existing ones, medical formulas they have developed from rainforest products, and even human genes they have discovered a particular use for. Lisa J. Raines, vice president for government affairs at the Industrial Biotechnology Association in Washington, D.C., believes scientists should have this right. Allowing scientists to have proprietorial interest in and to profit from their work, she says, is what has made the U.S. biotechnology industry so successful.

As you read, consider the following questions:

1. List two factors that the author says justify the right to patent biological products.
2. How does Raines say the example of insulin, used in the treatment of diabetics, supports her belief that scientists should be able to patent their products?
3. What does the author say will be the consequences if scientists are not allowed to patent their discoveries?

The biotechnology industry is an important new source of economic vitality for the United States. American scientists invented genetic engineering and American investors have funded the research and development (R&D) that enables the biotechnology industry to translate cutting-edge science into economic growth. As a result, the United States leads the world in the research, development, and manufacture of biotechnology products. In 1991, sales totaled $5.8 billion, an 18 percent increase over 1990, and net exports exceeded $600 million. The White House Council on Competitiveness projects that by the year 2000, biotechnology will be a $50-billion industry.

Thanks to its early lead, the U.S. biotechnology industry should claim a large share of that market. But without adequate legal protection for its innovations, the U.S. industry's early investment and progress will be worth little in global competition. The patent system, which should reward the achievements of biotechnology pioneers, is allowing intellectual pirates to copy innovative biotechnology products without penalty. Under current law, inventors cannot obtain effective patent protection for the products themselves, the processes by which they are created, or even the original materials used in these processes. The threat of domestic or foreign piracy undermines continued investment in R&D. Only statutory changes can protect the U.S. competitive edge in biotechnology.

Endangered Investments

One of the distinguishing characteristics of the biotechnology industry is the extraordinarily high level of investment in R&D. Since the inception of the biotechnology industry in the late 1970s, biotechnology companies have plowed at least $10 billion into long-term R&D programs; in 1991 alone, they spent $3.2 billion. They reinvested in R&D an average of 47 percent of the 1991 income generated by product sales—an average of $81,000 per employee. By comparison, pharmaceutical companies, traditionally considered the nation's most research-intensive, spent 14 percent of their 1991 income on R&D.

In such a research-intensive industry, the need to protect innovation is particularly urgent. Clearly, a pioneer company that commonly invests $100 million to $200 million to develop a new biopharmaceutical product must be assured that a competing company cannot pirate its intellectual achievements. And precisely because it is so expensive to innovate, other firms are highly motivated to find ways to short-cut the process.

Piracy is fairly easy to accomplish in biotechnology. For one thing, most scientific breakthroughs are routinely published in scientific journals, rather than being maintained as trade secrets. This aids research progress but makes it difficult to protect intellectual property. Once a journal has published an important scientific discovery, such as the genetic sequence that codes for a potentially important therapeutic protein, it is a fairly simple matter for other scientists to copy the product from this "recipe."

Biotechnology researchers can also use the equivalent of "reverse engineering" to reproduce competitors' inventions. When a company isolates or synthesizes a purified protein that appears to have therapeutic significance, it will begin preclinical and clinical trials of the substance to determine its usefulness in treating diseases. Once these studies begin, a competitor may obtain a sample of the material from a third party, such as a university where the trial is being conducted. It is then relatively easy to sequence the protein to determine its precise amino acid composition. This, in turn, enables the competitor to determine the gene sequence needed to synthesize the protein.

The tremendous cost of developing a new biotechnology product stands in stark contrast to the ease with which the product can be copied. Under these circumstances, clear and meaningful patent protection is essential.

Unpatentable Products

Modern biotechnology began with the first recombinant DNA experiment in 1973. But it was not until 1980—when the U.S. Supreme Court held that a genetically engineered microorganism was patentable—that biotechnology companies formed to commercialize recombinant DNA technology. This decision suggested that "everything under the sun made by man," including biotechnological inventions, was patentable.

Though genetically engineered microorganisms that produce useful proteins and enzymes are clearly patentable, the resulting biopharmaceutical products often are not. To be patentable, an invention must be *novel, non-obvious,* and *useful.* For instance, traditional pharmaceutical products are synthetic molecules, which easily meet the principal criteria of patentability. By contrast, a genetically engineered protein can be considered novel only if it was never known before it was isolated and purified. For example, tissue plasminogen activator, a naturally occurring protein that dissolves the coronary blood clots that cause heart attacks, was totally unknown before it was isolated by researchers using biotechnology techniques; it has been patented.

However, if the scientific literature reveals that the protein has previously been purified to some extent, even if it has not been definitively characterized, it may be ruled unpatentable for lack of novelty. The fact that previously available methods did not allow scientists to isolate enough of the protein for any practical use is considered irrelevant.

The case of insulin demonstrates the drawbacks inherent in trying to patent biotechnology products. Insulin was discovered in 1921, when scientists first removed a dog's pancreas, making the animal diabetic. By extracting canine insulin from the excised pancreas, they were able to treat the dog's diabetes. Several years later, other scientists isolated human insulin from human cadaver pancreases. All that these scientists knew was that they had a test tube containing a trace amount of human insulin. They didn't know what the chemical structure was or how to manufacture it.

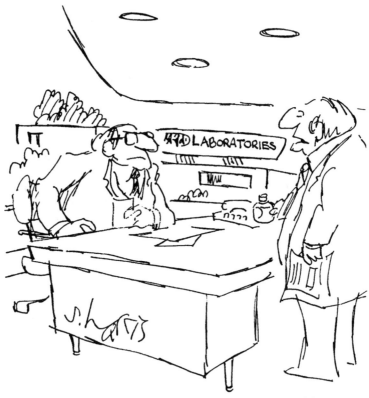

It's simple. If my breakthrough becomes the property of the company, I won't tell you what it is.

As a result, for more than 50 years after its discovery, human insulin was not available to treat diabetes. Instead, diabetics were forced to rely on animal insulin from the pancreases of slaughtered pigs and cows. This treatment was not always effective, since the immune system of some diabetics rejected the animal insulin as a foreign substance.

Nevertheless, the fact that human insulin had been isolated in the 1920s effectively barred the researchers who later made it possible to manufacture human insulin from obtaining a product patent. In 1951, Frederick Sanger succeeded in identifying the chemical structure and precise molecular weight of human insulin. This discovery won him the Nobel Prize, but it couldn't win him a patent. In 1979, David Goeddel synthesized recombinant human insulin, enabling patients the world over to gain access to the product they desperately needed. He couldn't get a product patent either.

Protecting the Process

In the absence of *product* patent protection, scientists can seek patent protection for the *process* used in making the product. Since genetic engineering is the only commercially feasible method for manufacturing human proteins, a patent on the recombinant manufacturing process can be tantamount to a product patent for biotechnology products, and many process patents have been granted. However, the ability of the biotechnology industry to obtain process-patent protection has been drastically circumscribed by the erroneous and inconsistent application of a Federal Circuit Court ruling.

In a 1985 decision, *In re Durden*, the U.S. Court of Appeals for the Federal Circuit (CAFC) denied a process patent. The appellants in *Durden* sought to patent a chemical process for making novel carbamate products from novel oxime starting materials. The applicants acknowledged that carbamates had previously been produced by reactions involving oxime compounds, but argued that the specific oximes used in the process as well as the carbamates produced were original.

The CAFC summarized the problem as follows: "The issue to be decided is whether a chemical process, otherwise obvious, is patentable because either or both the specific starting material employed and the product obtained are novel and non-obvious."

The court decided that the process could not be patented. It argued that the use of a different reaction material in an otherwise familiar process does not constitute a new reaction process. Even the applicants admitted that the results of this particular process were predictable. The court cautioned against applying *Durden* to processes involving other disciplines, but did not explicitly restrict its scope.

In the years since the *Durden* decision was issued, it has had a chilling effect on process-patent protection for the U.S. biotechnology industry. The U.S. Patent and Trademark Office (PTO) frequently cites *Durden* in denying patents to genetic engineering processes. A survey of the impact of *Durden*, commissioned by Genentech, a biotechnology company, shows that at least 60 percent of biotechnology product patents that do not have corresponding process patents can be directly linked to a *Durden* rejection.

The reasoning used in applying *Durden* to genetic engineering runs as follows: The basic process of genetic engineering is known. It consists of inserting a DNA molecule into a living cell so that the cellular machinery produces the specific protein encoded by the DNA molecule. Therefore, once a new DNA molecule has been invented, it is obvious that it can and should be used in a recombinant DNA process. Since non-obviousness is one of the three criteria for patentability, the process is not patentable.

The denial of process-claim protection is routine even if the starting materials are found by the patent examiner to be patentable in their own right. The *Durden* decision says, in effect, that it is obvious how to use an invention that never existed before. . . .

Other Precedents

In fact, there are other legal precedents directly in conflict with *Durden* that are far more readily applicable to biotechnology processes. The most significant of these is *In re Mancy*, a case involving a process using traditional culture techniques on a new bacterial strain to prepare an antibiotic. Even though the same basic culture techniques had been used on other strains to produce the antibiotic, using the process patent was upheld because of the patentability of the new strain.

It seems logical that *Mancy*, rather than *Durden*, should be applied to biotechnology cases. The process described in *Mancy* is analogous to the preparation of a desired protein by culturing a previously unknown, genetically engineered cell. Indeed, the reasoning in *Mancy* underlies the law for inventions in Europe and Japan, both of which have a long tradition of patenting process inventions that use patentable starting materials.

Why, then, does the PTO apply *Durden* rather than *Mancy* to genetic engineering cases? The reason appears to be that *Durden* and *Mancy* are characterized as two different kinds of process inventions. *Durden* deals with a *process of making* an end product, whereas *Mancy* refers to a *process of using* starting materials. Indeed, a more recent case, *In re Pleuddeman*, stated that "there is a real difference between a process of making and a process of using and the cases dealing with one involve different problems from cases dealing with the other."

Genetic engineering *uses* starting materials to *make* an end product, so that it may fairly be characterized as either a method of making or a method of using. By electing—for reasons that are unclear—to consider all biotechnology processes as method-of-making cases, the PTO has ruled that they should be governed by *Durden*. But the fundamental question is not whether they are making or using processes, but why these processes receive different treatment from the patent office.

Starting Materials Patents: An Alternative?

If an end product is not patentable because it lacks novelty (as in the case of insulin) and the genetic engineering process is not patentable because it is considered obvious under *Durden*, the inventor may nevertheless patent the starting materials. Obtaining a patent on a new DNA molecule or on the genetically engineered cell containing the inserted cell is relatively simple. However, unlike patents on products or processes, patents on starting materials fail to provide adequate protection from foreign competition.

A U.S. patent grants the right to prevent unauthorized parties from "making, using, or selling" the invention in the United States. If the patent is on an end product then not only can the product not be "made" in this country without the patentee's permission, it cannot be "sold" in this country, even if it is manufactured overseas and subsequently imported into the United States. Legislation enacted in 1988 extended this principle to process patents: It prohibits not only unauthorized domestic use of the process but also the import of foreign-manufactured products if a U.S.-patented process was used in making them.

But current law does not give starting-material patents the same enforcement rights. The rulings in two cases involving the California-based biotechnology company Amgen show that, although unauthorized domestic use of U.S.-patented starting materials constitutes patent infringement, the patent does not give a company the right to prevent other companies from using these starting materials overseas and then exporting the finished product to the United States.

Amgen pioneered the development of erythropoeitin (EPO), a hormone produced in the kidney that stimulates the production of red blood cells. Amgen holds a patent covering the gene that codes for EPO and the genetically engineered host cell into which the gene was inserted. Its patent on the EPO gene and host cell effectively prevents anyone else from making EPO in the United States, since these starting materials are essential for the production of EPO using genetic engineering techniques and genetic engineering is the only known way to make EPO in commercial quantities.

However, a Japanese company, Chugai Pharmaceutical, obtained the starting materials from a U.S. company, Genetics Institute. Genetics Institute's own use of these materials was held to be an act of infringement, and the company is now enjoined from further manufacture. The use of U.S.-patented starting materials by Genetic Institute's Japanese partner was *not* ruled to constitute infringement, even though the product is being manufactured for export to the United States. . . .

The phenomenal growth and competitive strength of the biotechnology industry can be directly attributed to the willingness of scientists and investors to devote their lives and savings to the discovery and implementation of scientific advances. By extending the scope of patent protection for their endeavors, the United States can reward their efforts and ensure the continued advancement of the biotechnology industry.

"When was it determined that the building blocks of life belonged not to God, humanity, or nature, but to patent holders?"

Biological Patents Affront Human Values

Andrew Kimbrell

Attorney Andrew Kimbrell is the author of *The Human Body Shop* and is policy director for the Foundation on Economic Trends in Washington, D.C. He believes that science goes too far when it tries to patent biological products and by-products. Although scientists deserve to be rewarded for their work, he says, they have no right to place an economic monopoly on such things as body parts, medical products derived from a patient's cells, and other such items. He asserts that such a crass, profit-centered action devalues human life to the extent that in the future people may see little distinction between a human and a machine.

As you read, consider the following questions:

1. What momentous patent issued in October 1991 has the potential of forever changing our perceptions about human life, according to the author? Do you agree with his perspective? Explain.
2. Does Kimbrell appear to be against patenting every biological product? If not, what kind of distinction does he draw?

From Andrew Kimbrell, "Patents Encroach upon the Body," *Crisis*, May 1993. Reprinted by permission of *Crisis* magazine, Box 1006, Notre Dame, IN 46556.

Over 200 years ago, Thomas Jefferson introduced America's first Patent Act. An amateur scientist himself, Jefferson was determined to ensure that "ingenuity should receive a liberal encouragement." In 1793, Congress enacted into law a proposal allowing inventors to patent "any new and useful art, machine, manufacture or composition of matter, or any new useful improvement [thereof]." As established by the 1793 law, a patent is a grant issued by the U.S. government giving the patent owner the sole right to make, use, or sell an invention within the United States during the term of the patent—generally 17 years. Whatever "machine, manufacture or composition of matter" invented—be it an airplane, computer, pesticide, or toaster—the patent provides a government-sanctioned monopoly to the inventor of the product. This is a financial reward for the inventor's ingenuity, designed to help the inventor recoup the time and expense spent in creating the new and "useful" invention.

For better or worse, the U.S. economy has been built on innovation rewarded by the patent system. Since 1793 over five million patents have been issued. Patents provided the profit trigger for the machine age in America. It's an American truism that behind each great discovery lies a patent.

But on October 29, 1991, the United States Patent and Trademark Office (PTO) issued a patent of a type never imagined by Jefferson and more startling than any of the millions that preceded it—a patent which represented a bold expansion of commerce into what can only be described as the "human body shop," and a major development in the industrialization of life. On that day, for the first time, the patent office granted patent rights to a naturally occurring part of the human body. Patent number 5,061,620 grants to Systemix Inc., of Palo Alto, California, corporate control of human bone marrow "stem cells" (stem cells being the progenitors of all types of cells in the blood). What makes the patent remarkable, and legally suspect, is that the patented cells were not any form of product or cell line. They had not been manipulated, engineered, or altered in any way. The PTO had never before allowed a patent on an unaltered part of the human body.

Patenting Human Cells

Stem cells, which are key to bone marrow transplants and other treatments designed to help a patient produce healthy blood, are difficult to isolate. Researchers at Systemix claim to have discovered a process that yields an unusually pure strain of stem cells. The Systemix process could represent a significant breakthrough in improving bone marrow transplants and in the developing of new genetic therapies for leukemia and a variety of other blood disorders—even for AIDS patients. What stunned

26

and outraged the scientific community was that the Systemix patent not only covers the process by which Systemix isolates human stem cells, but the stem cells themselves. "It really is outlandish to believe you can patent a stem cell," asserted Peter Quesenberry, medical affairs vice chairman of the Leukemia Society of America. "Where do you draw the line? Can you patent a hand?"

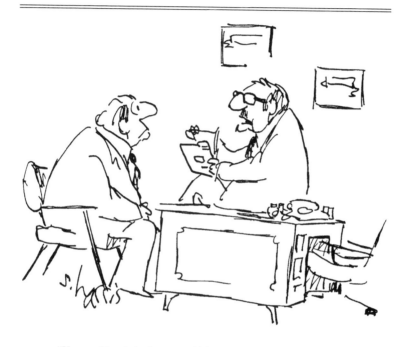

"Your problem is in the gene which makes antibodies, but since the Biophase Corp. now has a patent on that gene, I can't do anything for you."

If the stem cell patent survives an inevitable series of court challenges, every individual or institution which wishes to use stem cells for a commercial cure for diseases or disorders would have to come to a licensing agreement with Systemix. Systemix now has its own privately controlled monopoly on human stem cells. As ethicist Thomas Murray says, "they've invaded the commons of the body and claimed a piece of it for themselves."

The cell patent granted to Systemix has been accompanied by

patent applications even more astounding. On June 20, 1991, National Institutes of Health (NIH) researcher Craig Venter filed a 400-page patent application that would result in patent protection and ownership for 337 genes found in the human brain. This controversial application is seen by many in the scientific community as the first step in the patenting of all the 100,000 or more human genes. A few months after the first application, Venter applied for patents on 2,000 more brain genes fragments. This would represent patent ownership of roughly five percent of all human genes. . . .

Venter's patent claim has been aptly compared to a "quick and dirty land grab"—equivalent to attempting to claim large tracts of land in the hope that some of the acres contain oil or gold. Dr. James Watson, co-discoverer of the structure of DNA and former head of the $3 billion U.S. Human Genome Project, which is committed to mapping and sequencing each and every human gene, called the patent applications "sheer lunacy.". . . Then in July of 1992, Venter announced that he was leaving the NIH so as to establish his own gene-mapping institute with the help of $70 million from a venture capital fund. Locating and patenting genes has become big business.

Genetic Monopoly

Venter's patent application, and similar applications by other governmental and private corporations, create a unique and profoundly disturbing scenario. The entire human genome—the tens of thousands of genes that are our most intimate common heritage—will be owned by a handful of companies and governments. While the PTO up to now has not accepted Venter's applications, if his (and others) are accepted, a few government bureaucracies and powerful corporations will have a monopoly to make use of, or sell, all human genes. We will see the privatization of the genes that make up the human body—the corporate enclosure of our genetic commons.

Not surprisingly, the patenting of human cells and genes has led to massive legal and moral confusion. For example, one patient, John Moore, is suing the University of California for a share of the millions of dollars of profits being made on a cell line created from his spleen cells. The California Supreme Court denied his claim. Kevin O'Connor, a senior analyst at the U.S. Office of Technology Assessment (OTA), confesses that few have even begun to think through all the arguments on whether the human genome or combinations of genes and cells can be patented. Others are concerned about the potential patenting of human body parts including ultimately the entire human body. Derek Wood, head of the biotechnology patent office in London, comments:

This is clearly an area that is going to prove a pretty horren-
dous problem in the future. The difficulty is in deciding where
to draw the line between [patenting] genetic material and human beings per se. Until we have a specific case in front of us
we have to make some pretty delicate judgements.

Those delicate judgments will have to come sooner rather
than later. According to published reports, the European Patent
Office (EPO) has received patent applications which would
cover women who would be genetically engineered to produce
valuable human proteins in their mammary glands. The genetic
engineering of mammals (such as mice, cows, and sheep) to produce various valuable human proteins in their milk is underway
and has shown some success. The EPO patent applications
demonstrate that researchers want patent protection that would
include any women who would be genetically altered in a similar manner. In one reported instance, Grenada Biosciences of
Texas has applied to the EPO to patent genetically altered mammals created by Baylor College of Medicine in Houston, and
wants the patent to include both genetically altered animals and
humans. Brian Lucas, a British patent attorney who represented
Baylor College, has stated that the American patent attorneys
who wrote the Grenada/Baylor application that was submitted
to the EPO carefully crafted the application to include the coverage of women because "Someone, somewhere may decide
that humans are patentable." The attempt to patent a "pharm-
woman" who would produce valuable pharmaceutical products
in her breasts has stirred considerable controversy in Europe.
Paul Lamoye, the Belgian president of the European Green
Party, called the reports of the patent applications "chilling
news." He noted that "The fact that medical researchers and
biotech companies have the audacity to even apply for it is clear
evidence of the frightening direction this technology is taking."

How the Patenting of Life Came to Be

How could this be? How did our cells, genes, embryos, and
body parts become assignable commodities? How could living
things or parts of living things, including the human body, be
seen as patentable products indistinguishable from mechanical
or chemical products? When was it determined that the building
blocks of life belonged not to God, humanity, or nature, but to
patent holders? And perhaps most perplexing, when and how
was it determined that the historic question of the legal meaning of life was to be decided not by the people, but by the U.S.
Patent Office? The answers to these questions draw us back two
decades and to the very definition of a "slippery slope."

Working for General Electric in Schenectady, New York, in
1971, Indian microbiologist Ananda Mohan Chakrabarty set out

to develop a special kind of "bug" that would eat crude oil. Its central use would be to devour oil slicks created by tanker spills or similar disasters. Nature already had produced several strains of bacteria that had the propensity to digest different types of hydrocarbons in oil. All of these bacteria were from a family of bacteria known as Pseudomonas. Each of these bacteria had plasmids (auxiliary parcels of genes) which break up or "eat" oil. The trick was to somehow put them all together to get a "super," oil-eating bacteria. Chakrabarty performed this feat of genetic manipulation by fusing the genetic material from four types of Pseudomonas. Taking plasmids from three of the oil-eating bacteria, Chakrabarty transplanted them into the fourth, thereby creating a crossbred version with an enhanced appetite for oil.

Patents Harm Scientific Research

The point of patenting is to encourage the disclosure and utilization of information by assuring the protection of proprietary rights. . . . But the quest for proprietary rights is changing the norms and practices of science in commercially promising areas. . . . The preemptive nature of patents is skewing research directions, threatening to compromise the independence of the scientific research process. . . .

As scientists become prospectors and as maintaining proprietary rights becomes a priority, there are serious implications for the concept of science as a relatively disinterested source of neutral information.

Dorothy Nelkin, *The Scientist*, November 23, 1992.

In 1971, G.E. and Chakrabarty applied to the U.S. Patent and Trademark Office (PTO) for a patent on their genetically engineered microbe. After several years of review, the PTO declined the request. The agency rejected the Chakrabarty application on the premise that animate life forms are not patentable. PTO noted that, if either Jefferson or Congress had intended life to be patentable under the 1793 Act, they would say so in the law. The PTO also noted that, in the few instances in which life forms had been patented—certain asexually reproducing plants—it was not the Patent Office which authorized the patenting, but, rather, specially designed legislation passed by Congress.

G.E. and Chakrabarty appealed the Patent Office rejection to the Court of Customs and Patent Appeals (CCPA). To the shock of many, they won. In an historic opinion, the CCPA, in a three-to-two decision, reversed the decision by the Patent Office and held that Chakrabarty could patent the oil-eating microbe. For the first time in patent law history, a court had allowed the patenting of a life form. The opinion was direct: "the fact that microorganisms . . . are alive . . . [is] without legal significance." The legal distinction between living and non-living matter had been rejected. The court attempted to minimize its historic legal melding of animate with inanimate by noting that microorganisms were patentable because they are "more akin to inanimate chemical compositions such as reactants, reagents, and catalysts, than they are to horses and honeybees or raspberries and roses."

The PTO was not impressed by the CCPA's legal decision to patent life, even lowly life forms. It held to its original rejection of the G.E. patent, and appealed the CCPA decision to the Supreme Court. . . .By a five-to-four margin the Court upheld the patenting of life. Chakrabarty was to be granted his patent. . . .

All nine justices deciding the *Chakrabarty* case did agree on one thing. They specifically noted that this was a "narrow" case—one which did not affect the "future of scientific research." Chief Justice Warren Burger went out of his way to note that his decision in no way implicated "the gruesome parade of horribles," including the engineering and patenting of animals and man, cited in various amicus briefs. The complete failure by the Court to correctly assess the impacts of the *Chakrabarty* decision may go down as one of the most important judicial miscalculations in United States history.

"Enlightened" Decision?

The biotechnology industry heralded the Court's decision as "enlightened" and a "breakthrough." Others were not so sure. Ethicist and author Leon Kass summarized the concern of many:

> What is the principled limit to this beginning extension of the domain of private ownership and dominion over living nature? Is it not clear, if life is a continuum, there are no visible or clear limits, once we admit living species under the principle of ownership? The principle used in *Chakrabarty* says that there is nothing *in the nature of a being,* no, not even in the human patentor himself, that makes him immune to being patented. . . . To be sure, in general it makes sense to allow people to own what they have made, because they artfully made it. But to respect art without respect for life is finally contradictory.

The next decade was to prove correct both patenting proponents and opponents. Patenting *did* provide the trigger for a lucrative biotechnology industry. It also created the slippery slope feared by Kass and other ethicists.

In 1985, five years after the Court's historic decision, the PTO ruled that the *Chakrabarty* holding allowing the patenting of microbes could be extended to include the patenting of genetically engineered plants, seeds, and plant tissue. By 1987, the Reagan

31

Administration's patent "slippery slope" had turned into an icy precipice. On April 7 of that year, the Patent Office issued a ruling specifically extending the *Chakrabarty* ruling to include all "multicellular living organisms, including animals." The radical new patenting policy suddenly transformed a decision about patenting microbes into one allowing the patenting of all life forms on earth, including animals. The ruling meant that, if a researcher implants foreign cells or genes into an animal—for example, cancer cells into a mouse, or human growth genes into a pig—the genetically altered animal is considered a human invention under Jefferson's two-century-old definition of patentable "manufactures." The patented animal's legal status is no different from other manufactures such as automobiles or tennis balls.

For those concerned about the ethics of patenting life, the revolutionary 1987 ruling on the patentability of animals, signed by Donald J Quigg, Assistant Secretary and Commissioner of Patents and Trademarks, did have a silver lining. The PTO ruling excluded human beings from patentability. The restriction on patenting human beings was based on the Patent Office's interpretation of the Thirteenth Amendment of the Constitution, the anti-slavery amendment, which prohibits ownership of a human being. Unfortunately, there were several problems with the exemption of humans. For one, under the PTO's 1987 ruling, embryos and fetuses—human life forms not presently covered under Constitutional Thirteenth Amendment protection—*are* patentable, and so are genetically engineered human tissues, cells, and genes. In fact, a genetically engineered "human" kidney, cornea, arm or leg, or any other body part might well be patentable. As we have seen, even a genetically engineered woman who has been altered to produce a certain valuable pharmaceutical in her mammary glands may be patentable.

Patenting Animals

On April 12, 1988, the U.S. Patent Office issued the first patent on a living animal. The patent was issued to Harvard Professor Philip Leder and to Timothy A. Stewart of San Francisco for their creation of a transgenic mouse containing a variety of genes found in other species, including chickens and man. These foreign genes were engineered into the mouse's permanent germline in order to predispose it to developing cancer. The mouse was genetically engineered and designed to be a better research animal in which to test the virulence of various carcinogens.

In December 1992, and again in February 1993, five more animals were patented. There are now over 190 animal patents pending at the PTO. Many are for fish, cows, and pigs which have had human genes engineered into their permanent genetic codes in order to change size, skin consistency, reproduction, or other traits.

Now, as human cells are patented, and thousands of human brain genes are patent-pending, and almost 200 animals—many containing human genes—are lined up for patenting, we have an important perspective from which to survey the influence of the Supreme Court's ill-advised decision in *Chakrabarty*. The *Chakrabarty* decision has continued to extend up the chain of life. The patenting of microbes inexorably led to the patenting of plants, then animals, and, finally, human body elements. Most of the "gruesome parade of horribles" predicted by those opposing the 1980 patent decision have become, in dizzying rapidity, realities.

The distance traveled since the *Chakrabarty* decision in furthering the patenting of life can be highlighted by considering whether the Court, in 1980, would have ruled that life forms were patentable had the organism in question not been a lowly, ineffective, oil-eating bacteria, but a human embryo, or a genetically engineered chimpanzee, or the entire set of over 100,000 human genes. The answer, clearly, is *no*. The Supreme Court never would have ruled for the patenting of these other living organisms or human subparts. Any such decision would have led to an immediate uproar in the legal and ethical community. Yet, down the slippery slope of the last decade, just such an expansion of patenting has occurred. History has borne out bioethicist Robert Nelson's assessment of *Chakrabarty*: "It's a staggering decision. It removes one more barrier to the protection of human life. Good God, once you start patenting life, is there no stopping it?"

Now, as government agencies refine the legal and technical means to patent numerous life forms and untold thousands of humanity's genes and cells, we can only look with extreme trepidation at the future with regard to the patenting of life. There is little question that, unless stopped, the patenting juggernaut will continue to transgress into life in all its forms. As research continues in cell analysis and in the deciphering of the human genome, corporations and researchers will fight for patent ownership of commercially valuable genes and cells held to be the key to health, intelligence, or youth. As there are advances in reproductive technology, human embryos will be up for patent grabs. Animals with increasing numbers of human genes will be patented. Genetically engineered human body parts almost certainly will be patented. And, looking into the more distant future, perhaps a genetically altered human body itself may be patentable. As patenting continues, the legal distinction between life and machine, life and commodity will begin to vanish.

33

> *"My own preference remains to prohibit the purchase and sale of human tissue and cells for any purpose by anyone."*

Individuals Own All Rights to Their Body Cells

George J. Annas

In 1984 a physician-scientist patented a human cell line based on the cells he removed from the spleen of a leukemia patient. The patent made the doctor eligible to earn potentially millions of dollars on the cell line, which could be used in several kinds of important research. The patient was ignorant of the use to which his cells were being put, and he was not offered participation in the profits. In the following viewpoint, medical philosopher George J. Annas discusses his belief that this should not be allowed to happen. Annas is Utley Professor of Health Law and director of the Law, Medicine, and Ethics Program at Boston University Schools of Medicine and Public Health.

As you read, consider the following questions:

1. How did the courts assess patient John Moore's case against the physician who used his spleen cells? What does the author think about the court decisions?
2. "Informed consent" means that before patients are operated on, they are told exactly what will be done, and they understand and consent to this process. Does Annas think informed consent in a case such as Moore's would allow a doctor to ethically do what Moore's doctor did with Moore's spleen cells? Explain.

From George J. Annas, "Outrageous Fortune: Selling Other People's Cells," *Hastings Center Report*, November/December 1990. Reprinted with permission.

All men are mortal. John Moore is a man. Therefore, John Moore is mortal. This is uncontroversial. However, a cell line developed from John Moore's body, the "Mo" cell line, is described as immortal, and the lawsuit regarding John Moore's right to share in the profits produced by the cell line, although not immortal, may seem to be. A lower court previously rejected any claim Moore might have in a cell line developed from his diseased spleen, and an appeals court reversed this decision, holding that physicians and researchers could be held liable for conversion for using a patient's cells without permission. The Supreme Court of California has now partially reversed the appeals court ruling, and the litigation is likely to live on.

The Case of John Moore

In 1976 John Moore's physician, David W. Golde, recommended that Moore's spleen be removed as a treatment for hairy-cell leukemia. After surgeons removed the spleen, Golde and others took cells from it and cultured them into an "immortal" cell line that produced a variety of useful products. In 1984 this cell line was patented, and Golde and others will reap substantial profits from it. Moore alleges that he was never informed of any of this and never agreed to it. Assuming this is true, the questions presented are: (1) can Moore sue Golde for failure to disclose his pecuniary interest in producing a cell line from Moore's spleen as a breach of his fiduciary duty to the patient; and (2) can Moore sue the research companies and others who have used the cell line for a share in their profits from it? In a five-to-two opinion, Justice Panelli, writing for the California Supreme Court, answered the first question affirmatively, but refused to grant the patient any ownership interest in his cells after they had been removed from his body.

The California Supreme Court has been the nation's leader in the area of informed consent, deciding in 1972 that a physician had a "fiduciary" responsibility to the patient to disclose the nature of the proposed treatment, its alternatives, risks, and potential problems of recuperation. Past cases have all concentrated on the patient's choice and enhancing that choice by providing "material" information to the patient that might cause him or her to accept or reject the proposed treatment. The California Supreme Court has now ruled that the doctrine of informed consent requires a full financial disclosure because failure to make a financial disclosure is a violation of trust that undermines patient autonomy.

The goal is to protect patients from physicians whose judgment might be influenced by profit, and who might thus be in a conflict of interest position with their own patients. In the court's words:

[A] physician who treats a patient in whom he also has a research interest has potentially conflicting loyalties. . . . The possibility that an interest extraneous to the patient's health has affected the physician's judgment is something a reasonable patient would want to know in deciding whether to consent to a proposed course of treatment. It is material to the patient's decision and, thus, a prerequisite to informed consent.

This is not to say that physician-researchers are evil-minded, or intentionally advocate procedures not in their patients' best interests, only that "consciously or unconsciously . . . the physician's extraneous motivation may affect his judgment."

Selling Cells

The remaining defendants, the Regents of the University of California, a researcher, and two corporations, are not physicians and thus have no independent fiduciary duty to the patient. The appeals court had found them potentially liable for conversion of Moore's property interest in his cells. The California Supreme Court, however, reversed this holding. It gave three reasons: no case had ever decided that a patient had a continuing property interest in excised cells; California statutes drastically limit the patient's interest in excised cells; and the patented cell line is "both factually and legally distinct from the cells taken from Moore's body."

Probably because none of these reasons is terribly persuasive the court went on at length to discuss the public policy reasons that it believed supported the denial of Moore's property claim. Again there were three: a fair balancing of interests counsels against recognizing the claim; the legislature should solve this problem; and Moore's rights can be protected by a suit against the physician. Of these three, the centerpiece of the opinion is the first. The court essentially concluded that the biotechnology industry is both wonderful and fragile. Since it is wonderful, we must all do our part to foster it; and since it is fragile, we must protect it from harm.

Research on human cells plays a critical role in medical research. . . . Products developed through biotechnology that have already been approved for marketing in this country include treatments and tests for leukemia, cancer, diabetes, dwarfism, hepatitis-B, kidney transplant rejection, emphysema, osteoporosis, ulcers, anemia, infertility, and gynecological tumors, to name but a few. . . . The extension of conversion law into this area will hinder research by restricting access to the necessary raw materials.

In the court's flowery words, conversion (a strict liability tort that does not depend upon knowledge or motive) would threaten "to destroy the economic incentive to conduct important medical research . . . with every cell sample a researcher would purchase a ticket in the litigation lottery." On the other hand, denying Moore's property claim "will only make it more difficult for Moore to recover a highly theoretical windfall.". . . .

There are many ways to look at this case. As is clear from its text, the majority simply accepts the "Chicken Little" argument that if John Moore's property interests in his cells is upheld, the biotechnology industry's sky will fall and medical progress will suffer a major setback. In this regard the justices seem to have been blinded by science, and are unable or unwilling to distinguish it from commerce. . . . Even a "law and economics" approach would have required giving some value to Moore's cells, and would have insisted that it be taken into account as a cost of doing business in the biotechnology arena.

Let Patients Profit

Andrew Kimbrell: They patented Moore's cells and claimed the profits as their own. With *Diamond* [*v. Chakrabarty*], we have sanctioned the unholy alliance of the biotechnology industry and academia, of profits and science. And now people like John Moore will ask, "Why shouldn't I get my share?"

Lori Andrews: I agree. It seems unjustified to keep the patients out of the profit. People like to focus on the changes in biotechnology and the novelty of the science, but really, these possibilities have been around for years. People have sold blood. The first cell line, similar to John Moore's, was created in 1951. In the 1960s, Italian nuns donated their urine so that Pergonal, a fertility drug, could be made to help women have babies. The body has been a "factory" for quite a while. What's different now is the potential for commercialism. We're seeing it throughout medicine: the evolution of hospitals into profit centers and the increasing fees paid to certain physicians. Leon Rosenberg, dean of the Yale University School of Medicine, has observed that medical schools have moved from the classroom to the boardroom, from the *New England Journal of Medicine* to the *Wall Street Journal*, and, in my view, it's unfair to cut out the person who is contributing the most to this process.

"Forum: Sacred or for Sale?" *Harper's*, October 1990.

It is not necessarily wrong for courts to base their ultimate conclusions on their interpretation of public policy. On the other hand, courts have an obligation to analyze and struggle with novel questions of law as part of our common law tradition. It is thus very disappointing to see the majority simply ignore the insightful and powerful analysis of the appeals court on the issue of conversion. Instead of searching for possible analogies in the law that might illuminate the conflict, the court dismisses the conversion claim summarily with the statement that Moore is invoking "a tort theory originally used to determine whether the loser or the finder of a horse had the better title." This, and the fact that this is a case of first impression, seemed sufficient to the court to justify the conclusion that conversion should not apply.

This approach should be embarrassing to the court. Perhaps conversion is not the proper remedy; but the court makes no attempt to demonstrate why. Suppose Moore had a mare that was sick, and perhaps dying, and he asked his neighbor to take care of the horse so that it would not infect other animals on his farm. And suppose that the horse did not die, indeed, not only got better, but also had a prize colt. Instead of telling Moore about the recovery and the prize colt, assume the neighbor tells him that his mare has died, and then sells both the mare and the colt for $100,000. Should Moore be able to recover the $100,000 (less the cost of care) from the neighbor if he finds out that he has been lied to? The majority would probably say that because horses are involved, Moore should be able to recover; but if cells were involved, he should not. But without giving us a reason to distinguish cells from horses, we are left with a very unsatisfactory opinion.

Doctors and Profit

Even though most of the commentators on this case have concentrated on the conversion/property aspects of it, and have correctly argued that it is a major victory for the biotechnology industry, the most important aspect of the opinion deals with the expansion of the informed consent requirements based on the fiduciary nature of the doctor-patient relationship. The court has no problem with a biotechnology industry that breathlessly pursues profits: this is the way American business operates. But physicians are another matter altogether; when physicians are in a position to personally profit from their own treatment recommendations, they must disclose this financial or research aspect to their patient as part of informed consent. Of course this applies to Dr. Golde and John Moore. But it would also apply to physicians who recommend a procedure or treatment that will pay them more than an alternative treatment or procedure. Incentives need not be just financial; any "interest extraneous to the patient's health" that might affect the recommendation must be disclosed. Should informed consent now concentrate as much on the financial motives of the physician as on the nature of the proposed procedure? Should the physician's tax returns and percentage of income derived from the recommended procedure be part of informed consent?

The expansion of the informed consent doctrine in this manner, however, requires much more analysis than the court presents, and will undoubtedly be the subject for many cases in the future. When, for example, does the physician's personal interest in the treatment recommendation become so overwhelming as to *disqualify* the physician altogether as a potential advisor to the patient, and under what circumstances might a second, neutral opinion be required? In the organ and tissue business we already have two examples where ethical standards, although not law, counsel that even the appearance of a conflict of interest should disqualify the physician from making certain decisions. The first is that transplant surgeons should not be involved in the determination of death of a potential donor; and the second is that physicians who perform abortions should not get any rewards, financial or academic, from fetal tissue research.

Legislative Solutions

To paraphrase Leona Helmsley, the majority opinion concludes that "only the little people can't sell cells." This result will seem unfair to almost everyone; legislation seems both reasonable and likely. What should such legislation contain? If we are to permit commerce in body tissues, it seems unconscionable not to permit the individuals from whom these tissues are obtained to participate in the commerce. My own preference remains to prohibit the purchase and sale of human tissue and cells for any purpose by anyone. Alternatively, fairness and respect for persons require that we not only inform patients of the potential commercial applications of their organs, tissues, and cells, but also that we give them some opportunity to obtain reasonable compensation for this use. Since most tissues removed will not turn out to be valuable, and since paying even a small price for all of them may simply be a waste of money, perhaps the most reasonable thing to do is to provide that compensation shall be paid based on a standard fee schedule (e.g., 1 percent of gross sales), payment to be made either to the individual or to a nonprofit cell-line storage facility, the election to be made by the patient at the time of consent to the removal, and ratified at the time commercial value is determined.

This or some similar scheme will have to be adopted if we want to prevent physicians and researchers from being seen as simply opportunistic profit seekers. The law cannot remedy every "heartache and the thousand natural shocks that flesh is heir to," but it can serve quite adequately to craft reasonable commercial agreements that protect against "the slings and arrows of outrageous fortune" and are fair to all parties.

"We propose . . . a legal structure in which [property rights in] transplantable human tissue . . . can be created in new forms of tissue through the investment of labor."

Scientists Should Be Able to Own Cells They Have Altered

Margaret S. Swain and Randy W. Marusyk

In 1984 a doctor patented a cell line based on human spleen cells. In 1988 two researchers patented a mouse. In 1991 scientists working on the Human Genome Project attempted to patent genes even before they knew a purpose for them or had altered them. These and other cases have fed the controversy surrounding the intertwining of profit motive and biomedical research. In the following viewpoint, the authors propose a three-tiered classification of biomedical products to enable clear and ethical decisions to be made on their patentability. Margaret S. Swain holds a Ph.D. in neurochemistry from the University of Montreal, a law degree from McGill University, and is currently practicing biotechnology law in Ottawa, Canada. Randy W. Marusyk holds a M.Sc. in biochemistry, a law degree from McGill University, and is also practicing biotechnology law in Ottawa, Canada.

As you read, consider the following question:

1. Using the authors' recommended classification system, determine whether each of the three examples in the paragraph above would be patentable.

From Margaret S. Swain and Randy W. Marusyk, "An Alternative to Property Rights in Human Tissue," *Hastings Center Report*, September/October 1990. Reprinted with permission.

Recent developments in biotechnology involving human tissue are sweeping our interactions with this material well beyond the boundaries of existing law. Some of these developments allow profit-oriented companies to use human tissue to generate lucrative products such as drugs, diagnostic tests, and human proteins. The profits obtained elevate the monetary worth of certain types of human tissue, which until very recently has had little or no monetary value, to incalculable levels. Such changes require a society to reassess the present and future status of human tissue within the legal system.

As a free market society, we believe in the general principle of economic justice and attempt to render all individuals their economic due. Based on this general principle, some have argued for recognizing a limited form of property rights in human tissue, such that the profits can be shared amongst all who contribute to the development of the product, including the donor of the tissue. Still others have called for full recognition of property rights in human tissue such that organs and other tissues can be sold as a source of revenue for the donor.

This article investigates whether current ethical standards prohibiting a commercial market in transplantable organs and tissues can be maintained in a legal structure within which human tissue can also be used as a source to generate enormous profit. It is generally considered that the only options available are to recognize or not recognize property rights in human tissue. We propose instead a legal structure in which transplantable human tissue entails no property rights, but in which such rights can be created in new forms of tissue through the investment of labor. This structure will be applied to the facts of *Moore v. The Regents of the University of California* to illustrate how a claim based upon the recognition of property rights in human tissue would be decided.

Property Rights and the Body

Modern legal systems have consistently held that no property rights attach to the human body. This standard has been affirmed regardless of whether the human body was alive or not. However, the courts have recognized that a temporary right of possession may exist in a dead body in favor of an executor until proper disposal of the body has occurred. In *Pierce v. Proprietors of Swan Point Cemetery*, the Rhode Island Supreme Court held:

> Although . . . the body is not property in the usually recognized sense of the word, yet we may consider it as a sort of *quasi* property, to which certain persons may have rights, as they have duties to perform towards it, arising out of our common humanity. But the person having charge of it cannot be considered as the owner of it in any sense whatever; he holds

41

it only as a sacred trust for the benefit of all who may from family or friendship have an interest in it. . . .

This supposed "right" is not only a very limited possessory right (for purposes of a proper burial, etc.), exercisable only by the executor of an estate, but is recognized for a limited time; the "right" is extinguished upon burial or cremation.

Courts have also consistently refused to recognize any form of property rights in a living human body. This reflects society's moral abhorrence toward any form of slavery. When faced with a plaintiff seeking the recognition of property rights in his or her body, the courts have classified the action as a tort and analyzed the matter through this legal framework. Specific legislation, such as Congress's *National Organ Transplant Act*, builds upon this policy by explicitly prohibiting the *inter vivos* sale of many human organs.

Creating Property Rights Through Labor

How would this Lockean justification for the creation of property rights through labor apply to tissue permanently removed from the human body? Perhaps the following analogy will help us answer this question.

No one can claim exclusive property rights in information that is found in a common state, as this information is free for all to discover and utilize. . . . Such information can be used to create property through the cultivation of this information into a report. . . . Property rights are created when a person transforms this common information into a report; the particular collocation of words in which the reporter has communicated the information is where property rights are created by virtue of the *Copyright Act*.

Many parallels can be drawn between the information contained within a news report, and the utility contained within human matter, such as a cell line or particular sequence of genetic material.

Margaret S. Swain and Randy W. Marusyk, *Hastings Center Report*, September/October 1990.

Nevertheless, developments in biotechnology hold great promise for both the advancement of scientific knowledge and the improvement of human health, and this eventually requires the use of human tissue in research. Private industry will typically participate only in research from which it can generate profit to recoup its investment of time and money. However, to generate profit, it must be able to claim property rights in its research products. Thus, when private industry develops a commercial product—regardless if such products were generated through direct or indirect utilization of human tissue—it demands some form of proprietary protection (patents or trade secrets) for these products. Given society's ethical standard of forbidding the recognition of property rights in human tissue, the question is how these standards can be maintained while allowing private industry to secure property rights in their inventions that directly or indirectly involve human tissue.

We can identify three distinct levels to classify the substance that makes up the whole human being. The first level is that of the person and persona. The second is that of a functional bodily unit, such as blood, an organ, or cell, which can be transplanted into another person and carry out its function in the same capacity it did in its originator. At a third level, something must be produced from the human material, such as a cell line or cloned genetic material, for it to become useful. It is through the labor of cultivating the tissue that the laborer could claim property rights in the final product.

The Level of Person

According to Kantian philosophy, it is imperative that a legal system distinguish natural persons from things. The concept of free will differentiates human beings from mere objects, and dictates that human beings receive nothing less than full human dignity. If free will is recognized as the basis of moral rights, then it is this free will that allows humans to exercise control over objects.

The legal recognition of property rights in the pecuniary value of one's name, voice, appearance, and personal features may appear contrary to this basic philosophy. However, these "rights of publicity" are property rights that attach to *the concept* of a human entity and not directly to the human body itself. Such rights disappear upon the death of the natural person though the corpse may continue to exist, as exemplified in *Lugosi v. Universal Pictures* where it was questioned whether the persona of a movie actor—a proprietary right—could be passed on to his heirs. The court held that there did exist a right in an actor's name and likeness but that this right did not survive the actor.

In this first level, then, the legal structure should view the human body in its entirety, including the persona. This level represents the most complex sum of the parts (that is, organs, tissue, proteins, genetic material, etc.) and could not be attained by any one of the parts independently. Although each of the parts are very similar, if not identical, from person to person, the *sum total collection* of these parts creates a unique individual. As long as the parts remain within that person, they serve the function of that total and hence fall under the classification of property

43

rights for that total, viz., the "rights of publicity." However, once a part is removed from the total in such a way that it no longer functionally serves its original possessor, it would fall within the second level of the legal structure.

Res Nullius

The second level is constituted by functional bodily units capable of being transplanted. Upon removal from a person, human bodily material would be statutorily or judicially deemed *res nullius*; it would become a corporeal moveable owned by no one. If tissue is removed for transplantation into another person, the tissue would lose its *res nullius* status once the transplant was complete. Additionally, by having extracted tissue pass through the *res nullius* categorization, a donor would be prohibited from legally reclaiming rights in his transplanted tissue at some later date.

Under the classical definition of *res nullius*, ownership would be acquired by the first person who took possession of the tissue. However, for the purpose of transplantation, the legal system could deem those in possession of the excised tissue—physicians, nurses, or tissue transporters—as being possessors "in trust" of the tissue until the transplant was complete. During this period, the tissue would be classified as *trust res nullius;* a thing owned by nobody but held in trust for a recipient.

A categorical distinction must be made regarding tissue that is permanently removed from the body as opposed to tissue that is temporarily removed with the intention of having it subsequently become part of the same person. A temporary removal may come about by an unintentional event such as the accidental amputation of a limb or by an intentional act such as the storage of blood for use in future surgery. In these situations, the patient would be both the donor and the recipient; the person in possession during the interim would be the trustee.

Some companies, such as those that concentrate bone marrow or blood factors, may be concerned that their products would fall under the second level of classification, prohibiting them from being able to protect their products for lack of property rights. These products are types of human tissue that have been temporarily removed with the intention of transplantation into another body. Furthermore, such products are composed of tissue maintained in its original form. However, these products could be protected through other means, such as the doctrine of unjust enrichments arising for a service performed.

The benefit of declaring a functional unit of bodily material *res nullius* is that this material will continue to serve humankind (for example, organ transplant and blood transfusion) under a traditional altruistic spirit without becoming a marketable commodity, as could occur if property rights were to be recognized in it. Furthermore, isolating human transplantable tissue within its own classification would serve to protect its status in the future where the unknowns of technological development might threaten its status. Tissue that is *permanently* removed from a body, however, would fall under a third level of classification.

Res Communes Omnium

A third level would deem permanently removed human tissue as *res communes omnium*: things that by natural law are the common property of all humans. This classification would allow human material to be used in conjunction with high technology to generate property rights in the product. However, only after something is produced from tissue deemed *res communes omnium* could property rights be created in that thing. A key distinction between matter deemed *res communes omnium* and *res nullius* is that the latter need not be transformed in any way to be useful to humankind: it functions in much its original form.

This view of property reflects the philosophical justification of property expounded by John Locke's labor theory. Locke's justification rested upon two basic assumptions: A person has the right to maintain his life; and, God has provided us with the means to carry out this maintenance. The entire world is a common resource given by God to all persons to maintain themselves. These resources are the raw materials from which useful things are made through a person's labor. Since the labor is part of the person himself, as soon as the person mixes his labor with these raw materials to create a new product, he creates something that belongs only to him and nobody else. Locke stated that:

> It being by him removed from the common state Nature placed it in, it hath by this labour something annexed to it that excludes the common right of other men. For this labour being the unquestionable property of the labourer, no man but he can have a right to what that is once joined to. . . .

Thus the creation of a new thing through merging that thing with one's labor results in property that that person alone has the right to own; this is the case regardless if the labor is performed directly by the person, a servant under that person's control, or an animal (or machine) under that person's ownership. . . .

Scientists could justify a claim for ownership in a cell line, and products generated therefrom, much in the same way that a news gathering agency claims rights in the news that it has collected and collocated. As stated by the U.S. Supreme Court in the case of *International News Service v. The Associated Press*:

> Not only do the acquisition and transmission of news require elaborate organization and a large expenditure of money, skill,

and effort; not only has it an exchange value to the gatherer, dependent chiefly upon its novelty and freshness, the regularity of the service, its reputed reliability and thoroughness, and its adaptability to the public needs; but also, as is evident, the news has an exchange value to one who can misappropriate it.

Thus, the transformation of this information into a news report or the transformation of a cell's genetic material into a viable product (for example, via cloning) would, through labor, produce a new thing capable of being owned. The newspaper article is property under the *Copyright Act*, whereas the new genetic material would enjoy property rights under the *Patent Act* or trade secret law. . . .

The *Moore* Case

How might this structure be applied to the facts of *Moore*, a case involving nonconsensual use of the plaintiff's cancerous spleen cells to develop lucrative pharmaceutical products? The crux of this dispute concerned whether the plaintiff held personal property rights in the tissue and substances of his body and, if so, whether these rights were breached when the defendant converted this tissue for commercial profit.

The first level of the structure is not applicable to the facts of *Moore*. A persona attaches to the whole person; these proprietary rights would not apply to a mere part of a person such as a cell or a strand of DNA. The second level pertains to tissue destined for transplantation and is also not applicable to the facts of the *Moore* case.

As Moore's spleen and blood were removed with the intention of being permanently removed, this tissue would be classified as *res communes omnium*. This classification would not recognize the existence of property rights in human tissue, yet it would allow laborers to generate property rights through work—justified by a Lockean analysis. This would deny Moore any form of remuneration based upon property rights in his tissue. However, it would not deny the plaintiff the right to seek recourse through causes of actions independent of the need to have property rights in the human body.

Legally classifying the substances that make up humans into three distinct levels as we have suggested would thus allow us to preserve society's present ethical standards with regard to the transplantation of human tissue as an altruistic donation while at the same time allowing laborers to secure property rights in their inventions. Such a classification would, moreover, allow the legal system expressly to address our intuitive sense that while we each partake of universals of physiology, as unique personae we are more than the mere aggregation of our interchangeable parts.

"Randomized [human] trials are . . . the most scientifically sound and ethically correct means of evaluating new therapies."

Randomized Human Experimentation Is Essential to Biomedical Research

Eugene Passamani

Many experts believe that human subjects are essential to scientific research, particularly research to evaluate medical techniques and medicines. A *randomized clinical trial* is research conducted on real patients rather than laboratory subjects, and in which the subjects (patients) are selected by chance. This, researchers hope, eliminates the biased results that might occur if too many of the subjects shared similar traits. In the following viewpoint, Dr. Eugene Passamani of the National Heart, Lung, and Blood Institute argues that such trials are the only way to judge the true efficacy of certain treatments and that they are ethical as long as the patients have had the opportunity to give informed consent.

As you read, consider the following questions:

1. How does Passamani think randomized clinical trials can prevent such tragedies as the thalidomide debacle of the 1950s and 1960s?
2. Under what kinds of circumstances does the author believe the use of human subjects can be unethical?

Adapted from Eugene Passamani, "Clinical Trials—Are They Ethical?" *The New England Journal of Medicine*, vol. 324, no. 22, May 30, 1991. (The original article contains references and graphics not reproduced here.) Reprinted with permission.

Biomedical research leads to better understanding of biology and ultimately to improved health. Physicians have for millenniums attempted to understand disease, to use this knowledge to cure or palliate, and to relieve attendant suffering. Improving strategies for prevention and treatment remains an ethical imperative for medicine. Until very recently, progress depended largely on a process of carefully observing groups of patients given a new and promising therapy; outcome was then compared with that previously observed in groups undergoing a standard treatment. Outcome in a series of case patients as compared with that in nonrandomized controls can be used to assess the treatment of disorders in which therapeutic effects are dramatic and the pathophysiologic features are relatively uncomplicated, such as vitamin deficiency or some infectious diseases. Observational methods are not very useful, however, in the detection of small treatment effects in disorders in which there is substantial variability in expected outcome and imperfect knowledge of complicated pathophysiologic features (many vascular disorders and most cancers, for example). The effect of a treatment cannot easily be extracted from variations in disease severity and the effects of concomitant treatments. Clinical trials have thus become a preferred means of evaluating an ever increasing flow of innovative diagnostic and therapeutic maneuvers. The randomized, double-blind clinical trial is a powerful technique because of the efficiency and credibility associated with treatment comparisons involving randomized concurrent controls.

The modern era of randomized trials began in the early 1950s with the evaluation of streptomycin in patients with tuberculosis. Since that time trial techniques and methods have continuously been refined. In addition, the ethical aspects of these experiments in patients have been actively discussed.

In what follows I argue that randomized trials are in fact the most scientifically sound and ethically correct means of evaluating new therapies. There is potential conflict between the roles of physician and physician-scientist, and for this reason society has created mechanisms to ensure that the interests of individual patients are served should they elect to participate in a clinical trial.

Clinical Research

The history of medicine is richly endowed with therapies that were widely used and then shown to be ineffective or frankly toxic. Relatively recent examples of such therapeutic maneuvers include gastric freezing for peptic ulcer disease, radiation therapy for acne, MER-29 (triparanol) for cholesterol reduction, and thalidomide for sedation in pregnant women. The 19th century was even more gruesome, with purging and bloodletting. The reasons for this march of folly are many and include, perhaps most importantly, the lack of complete understanding of human biology and pathophysiology, the use of observational methods coupled with the failure to appreciate substantial variability between patients in their response to illness and to therapy, and the shared desire of physicians and their patients for cure or palliation.

Chance or bias can result in the selection of patients for innovative treatment who are either the least diseased or the most severely affected. Depending on the case mix, a treatment that has no effect can appear to be effective or toxic when historical controls are used. With the improvement in diagnostic accuracy and the understanding of disease that has occurred with the passage of time, today's patients are identified earlier in the natural history of their disease. Recently selected case series therefore often have patients who are less ill and an outcome that is considerably better than that of past case series, even without changes in treatment.

Human Trials Are Safe

"The word 'experimental' may frighten people," says Lawrence Friedman, M.D., chief of the Clinical Trials Branch of the National Heart, Blood, and Lung Institute in Bethesda, Md. "But by the time a treatment gets to the point where humans are used, short-term safety and effectiveness are established. What we're looking for at this stage is evidence that the new treatment has advantages over existing, approved therapies."

Sue Berkman, *Good Housekeeping*, August 1991.

Randomization tends to produce treatment and control groups that are evenly balanced in both known and unrecognized prognostic factors, which permits a more accurate estimate of treatment effect in groups of patients assigned to experimental and standard therapies. A number of independent randomized trials with congruent results are powerful evidence indeed.

A physician's daily practice includes an array of preventive, diagnostic, and therapeutic maneuvers, some of which have been established by a plausible biologic mechanism and substantial evidence from randomized clinical trials (e.g., the use of betablockers, thrombolytic therapy, and aspirin in patients with myocardial infarction). It is unlikely that our distant descendants in medicine will discover that we late-20th-century physicians were wrong in these matters. However, new therapeutic maneuvers that have not undergone rigorous assessment may well turn out to be ineffective or toxic. Every therapy adopted by common consent on the basis of observational studies and plausible mechanism, but without the benefit of randomized studies, may be categorized by future physicians as useless or worse. Physicians are aware of the fragility of the evidence supporting many common therapies, and this is why properly performed randomized clinical trials have profound effects on medical practice. The scientific importance of randomized, controlled trials is in safeguarding current and future patients from our therapeutic passions. Most physicians recognize this fact.

Like any human activity, experimentation involving patients can be performed in an unethical and even criminal fashion. Nazi war crimes led to substantial efforts to curb abuse, beginning with the Nuremberg Code and the Helsinki Declaration and culminating in the promulgation of clearly articulated regulations in the United States and elsewhere. There are abuses more subtle than those of the Gestapo and the SS. Involving patients in experiments that are poorly conceived and poorly executed is unethical. Patients who participate in such research may incur risk without the hope of contributing to a body of knowledge that will benefit them or others in the future. The regulations governing human experimentation are very important, as is continuing discussion and debate to improve the scientific and ethical aspects of this effort.

Clinical Experimentation

Several general features must be part of properly designed trials. The first is informed consent, which involves explicitly informing a potential participant of the goals of the research, its potential benefits and risks, the alternatives to participating, and the right to withdraw from the trial at any time. Whether informed consent is required in all trials has been debated. I believe that patients must always be aware that they are part of an experiment. Second, a state of clinical equipoise must exist. Clinical equipoise means that on the basis of the available data, a community of competent physicians would be content to have their patients pursue any of the treatment strategies being tested in a randomized trial, since none of them have been clearly established as preferable. The chief purpose of a data-monitoring committee is to stop the trial if the accumulating data destroy the state of clinical equipoise—that is, indicate efficacy or suggest toxicity. Finally, the trial must be designed as a critical test of the therapeutic alternatives being assessed. The question must be clearly articulated, with carefully defined measures of outcome; with realistic estimates of sample size, including probable event rates in the control group and a postulated and plausible reduction in the event rates in the treatment group; with Type I and II errors specified; and with subgroup hypotheses clearly stated if appropriate. The trial must have a good chance of settling an open question.

Experimentation in the clinic by means of randomized, controlled clinical trials has been periodically attacked as violating the covenant between doctor and patient. Critics have charged that physicians engaged in clinical trials sacrifice the interests of the patient they ask to participate to the good of all similarly affected patients in the future. The argument is that physicians have a personal obligation to use their best judgment and recommend the "best" therapy, no matter how tentative or inconclusive the data on which that judgment is based. Physicians must play their hunches. According to this argument, randomized clinical trials may be useful in seeking the truth, but carefully designed, legitimate trials are unethical and perhaps even criminal because they prevent individual physicians from playing their hunches about individual patients. Therefore, it is argued, physicians should not participate in such trials.

It is surely unethical for physicians to engage knowingly in an activity that will result in inferior therapy for their patients. It is also important that the community of physicians be clear in distinguishing between established therapies and those that are promising but unproved. It is this gulf between proved therapies and possibly effective therapies (all the rest) that defines the ethical and unethical uses of randomized clinical trials. Proved therapies involve a consensus of the competent medical community that the data in hand justify using a treatment in a given disorder. It is this consensus that defines an ethical boundary. The physician-investigator who asks a patient to participate in a randomized, controlled trial represents this competent medical community in asserting that the community is unpersuaded by existing data that an innovative treatment is superior to standard therapy. Arguments that a physician who believes that such a treatment *might* be useful commits an unethical act by randomizing patients are simply wrong. Given the history of promising but discarded therapies, hunches about potential effectiveness are not the ideal currency of the patient-doctor interchange.

Lest readers conclude that modern hunches are more accurate than older ones, I have selected an example from the current cardiovascular literature that reveals the problems inherent in relying on hunches to the exclusion of carefully done experiments.

The Cardiac Arrhythmia Suppression Trial

Sudden death occurs in approximately 300,000 persons in the United States each year and is thus a problem worthy of our best efforts. In the vast majority of cases the mechanism is ventricular fibrillation superimposed on a scarred [heart muscle]. . . . It had been established that a variety of antiarrhythmic drugs can suppress [some irregular heart contractions]. Accordingly, physicians had the hunch that suppressing [them] in the survivors of myocardial infarction [heart attacks] would reduce the incidence of . . . sudden death.

The Cardiac Arrhythmia Suppression Trial (CAST) investigators decided to test this hypothesis in a randomized, controlled trial. They sought survivors of myocardial infarction who had frequent [irregular heart contractions] on electrocardiographic recordings. . . . The trial had to be stopped prematurely because of an unacceptable incidence of sudden death in the treatment group. During an average follow-up of 10 months, 56 of 730 patients (7.7 percent) assigned to active drug and 22 of 725 patients (3.0 percent) assigned to placebo died. Clinical equipoise was destroyed by this striking effect. It is quite unlikely that observational (nonrandomized) methods would have detected this presumably toxic effect.

The CAST trial was a major advance in the treatment of patients with coronary disease and ventricular arrhythmia. It clearly revealed that the hunches of many physicians were incorrect. The trial's results are applicable not only to future patients with coronary disease and ventricular arrhythmia but also to the patients who participated in the study. By randomizing, investigators ensured that half the participants received the better therapy—in this case placebo—and, contrary to intuition, most of them ultimately received the better therapy after the trial ended prematurely and drugs were withdrawn.

To summarize, randomized clinical trials are an important element in the spectrum of biomedical research. Not all questions can or should be addressed by this technique; feasibility, cost, and the relative importance of the issues to be addressed are weighed by investigators before they elect to proceed. Properly carried out, with informed consent, clinical equipoise, and a design adequate to answer the question posed, randomized clinical trials protect physicians and their patients from therapies that are ineffective or toxic. Physicians and their patients must be clear about the vast gulf separating promising and proved therapies. The only reliable way to make this distinction in the face of incomplete information about pathophysiology and treatment mechanism is to experiment, and this will increasingly involve randomized trials. The alternative—a retreat to older methods—is unacceptable.

Physicians regularly apply therapies tested in groups of patients to an individual patient. The likelihood of success in an individual patient depends on the degree of certainty evident in the group and the scientific strength of the methods used. We owe patients involved in the assessment of new therapies the best that science and ethics can deliver. Today, for most unproved treatments, that is a properly performed randomized clinical trial.

"The randomized clinical trial routinely asks physicians to sacrifice the interests of their particular patients for the sake of the study."

Randomized Human Experimentation Is Not Essential to Biomedical Research

Samuel Hellman and Deborah S. Hellman

Deborah S. Hellman of Harvard University and Samuel Hellman of the University of Chicago, authors of the following viewpoint, contend that human trials of medical treatments are unnecessary and often unethical. While the physician's primary purpose should be to help the patient, they say, clinical trials make the research of paramount importance and the patient's welfare only secondary.

As you read, consider the following questions:

1. How do the authors distinguish between the role of the scientist and the role of the physician? Why do they think the two roles are often incompatible?
2. Do the authors think that research involving eager volunteers, such as AIDS patients anxious to try an unproven but potentially curative drug, are acceptable? Explain their position.
3. What alternatives do the Hellmans suggest to randomized clinical trials?

Adapted from Samuel Hellman and Deborah S. Hellman, "Of Mice but Not Men," *The New England Journal of Medicine*, vol. 324, no. 22, May 30, 1991. (The original article contains references and graphics not reproduced here.) Reprinted with permission.

As medicine has become increasingly scientific and less accepting of unsupported opinion or proof by anecdote, the randomized controlled clinical trial has become the standard technique for changing diagnostic or therapeutic methods. The use of this technique creates an ethical dilemma. Researchers participating in such studies are required to modify their ethical commitments to individual patients and do serious damage to the concept of the physician as a practicing, empathetic professional who is primarily concerned with each patient as an individual. Researchers using a randomized clinical trial can be described as physician-scientists, a term that expresses the tension between the two roles. The physician, by entering into a relationship with an individual patient, assumes certain obligations, including the commitment always to act in the patient's best interests. As Leon Kass has rightly maintained, "the physician must produce unswervingly the virtues of loyalty and fidelity to his patient." Though the ethical requirements of this relationship have been modified by legal obligations to report wounds of a suspicious nature and certain infectious diseases, these obligations in no way conflict with the central ethical obligation to act in the best interests of the patient medically. Instead, certain nonmedical interests of the patient are preempted by other social concerns.

Role of Scientist

The role of the scientist is quite different. The clinical scientist is concerned with answering questions—i.e., determining the validity of formally constructed hypotheses. Such scientific information, it is presumed, will benefit humanity in general. The clinical scientist's role has been well described by Dr. Anthony Fauci, director of the National Institute of Allergy and Infectious Diseases, who states the goals of the randomized clinical trial in these words: "It's not to deliver therapy. It's to answer a scientific question so that the drug can be available for everybody once you've established safety and efficacy." The demands of such a study can conflict in a number of ways with the physician's duty to minister to patients. The study may create a false dichotomy in the physician's opinions: according to the premise of the randomized clinical trial, the physician may only know or not know whether a proposed course of treatment represents an improvement; no middle position is permitted. What the physician thinks, suspects, believes, or has a hunch about is assigned to the "not knowing" category, because knowing is defined on the basis of an arbitrary but accepted statistical test performed in a randomized clinical trial. Thus, little credence is given to information gained beforehand in other ways or to information accrued during the trial but without the required statistical degree of assurance that a difference is not due to chance. The randomized clinical trial also prevents the treatment technique from being modified on the basis of the growing knowledge of the physicians during their participation in the trial. Moreover, it limits access to the data as they are collected until specific milestones are achieved. This prevents physicians from profiting not only from their individual experience, but also from the collective experience of the other participants.

Conflicting Ethical Demands

The randomized clinical trial requires doctors to act simultaneously as physicians and as scientists. This puts them in a difficult and sometimes untenable ethical position. The conflicting moral demands arising from the use of the randomized clinical trial reflect the classic conflict between rights-based moral theories and utilitarian ones. The first of these, which depend on the moral theory of Immanuel Kant (and seen more recently in neo-Kantian philosophers, such as John Rawls), asserts that human beings, by virtue of their unique capacity for rational thought, are bearers of dignity. As such, they ought not to be treated merely as means to an end; rather, they must always be treated as ends in themselves. Utilitarianism, by contrast, defines what is right as the greatest good for the greatest number—that is, as social utility. This view, articulated by Jeremy Bentham and John Stuart Mill, requires that pleasures (understood broadly, to include such pleasures as health and well-being) and pains be added together. The morally correct act is the act that produces the most pleasure and the least pain overall.

A classic objection to the utilitarian position is that according to that theory, the distribution of pleasures and pains is of no moral consequence. This element of the theory severely restricts physicians from being utilitarians, or at least from following the theory's dictates. Physicians must care very deeply about the distribution of pain and pleasure, for they have entered into a relationship with one or a number of individual patients. They cannot be indifferent to whether it is these patients or others that suffer for the general benefit of society. Even though society might gain from the suffering of a few, and even though the doctor might believe that such a benefit is worth a given patient's suffering (i.e., that utilitarianism is right in the particular case), the ethical obligation created by the covenant between doctor and patient requires the doctor to see the interests of the individual patient as primary and compelling. In essence, the doctor-patient relationship requires doctors to see their patients as bearers of rights who cannot be merely used for the greater good of humanity.

The randomized clinical trial routinely asks physicians to sacrifice the interests of their particular patients for the sake of the

55

study and that of the information that it will make available for the benefit of society. This practice is ethically problematic. Consider first the initial formulation of a trial. In particular, consider the case of a disease for which there is no satisfactory therapy —for example, advanced cancer or the acquired immunodeficiency syndrome (AIDS). A new agent that promises more effectiveness is the subject of the study. The control group must be given either an unsatisfactory treatment or a placebo. Even though the therapeutic value of the new agent is unproved, if physicians think that it has promise, are they acting in the best interests of their patients in allowing them to be randomly assigned to the control group? Is persisting in such an assignment consistent with the specific commitments taken on in the doctor-patient relationship? As a result of interactions with patients with AIDS and their advocates, [T.C.] Merigan recently suggested modifications in the design of clinical trials that attempt to deal with the unsatisfactory treatment given to the control group. The view of such activists has been expressed by Rebecca Pringle Smith of Community Research Initiative in New York: "Even if you have a supply of compliant martyrs, trials must have some ethical validity.". . .

Placebo Ethics

The ethical aspects of withholding a possible life-saving medication from one-half of a population to "prove" therapeutic efficacy are obviously critical. Indeed, one may justifiably conclude that, in the case of a serious, life-threatening situation, *any* testing of a potential therapeutic agent must be performed *without* the use of a corresponding placebo group.

Roger P. Maickel, *Priorities*, Fall 1990.

Even if it is ethically acceptable to begin a study, one often forms an opinion during its course—especially in studies that are impossible to conduct in a truly double-blinded fashion— that makes it ethically problematic to continue. The inability to remain blinded usually occurs in studies of cancer or AIDS, for example, because the therapy is associated by nature with serious side effects. Trials attempt to restrict the physician's access to the data in order to prevent such unblinding. Such restrictions should make physicians eschew the trial, since their ability to act in the patient's best interests will be limited. Even supporters of randomized clinical trials, such as Merigan, agree that interim findings should be presented to patients to ensure that no one receives what seems an inferior treatment. Once physicians have formed a view about the new treatment, can they continue randomization? If random assignment is stopped, the study may be lost and the participation of the previous patients wasted. However, if physicians continue the randomization when they have a definite opinion about the efficacy of the experimental drug, they are not acting in accordance with the requirements of the doctor-patient relationship. Furthermore, as their opinion becomes more firm, stopping the randomization may not be enough. Physicians may be ethically required to treat the patients formerly placed in the control group with the therapy that now seems probably effective. To do so would be faithful to the obligations created by the doctor-patient relationship, but it would destroy the study.

"Informed Consent"

To resolve this dilemma, one might suggest that the patient has abrogated the rights implicit in a doctor-patient relationship by signing an informed-consent form. We argue that such rights cannot be waived or abrogated. They are inalienable. The right to be treated as an individual deserving the physician's best judgment and care, rather than to be used as a means to determine the best treatment for others, is inherent in every person. This right, based on the concept of dignity, cannot be waived. What of altruism, then? Is it not the patient's right to make a sacrifice for the general good? This question must be considered from both positions—that of the patient and that of the physician. Although patients may decide to waive this right, it is not consistent with the role of a physician to ask that they do so. In asking, the doctor acts as a scientist instead. The physician's role here is to propose what he or she believes is best medically for the specific patient, not to suggest participation in a study from which the patient cannot gain. . . .

Moreover, even if patients could waive this right, it is questionable whether those with terminal illness would be truly able to give voluntary informed consent. Such patients are extremely dependent on both their physicians and the health care system. Aware of this dependence, physicians must not ask for consent, for in such cases the very asking breaches the doctor-patient relationship. Anxious to please their physicians, patients may have difficulty refusing to participate in the trial the physicians describe. The patients may perceive their refusal as damaging to the relationship, whether or not it is so. Such perceptions of coercion affect the decision. Informed-consent forms are difficult to understand, especially for patients under the stress of serious illness for which there is no satisfactory treatment. The forms are usually lengthy, somewhat legalistic, complicated, and confusing, and they hardly bespeak the compassion expected of the

57

medical profession. It is important to remember that those who have studied the doctor-patient relationship have emphasized its empathetic nature. [W.T. Longcope writes, the] "relationship between doctor and patient partakes of a peculiar intimacy. It presupposes on the part of the physician not only knowledge of his fellow men but sympathy. . . . This aspect of the practice of medicine has been designated as the art; yet I wonder whether it should not, most properly, be called the essence." How is such a view of the relationship consonant with random assignment and informed consent? The Physician's Oath of the World Medical Association affirms the primacy of the deontologic view of patients' rights: "Concern for the interests of the subject must always prevail over the interests of science and society.". . .

Find Other Methods

It is fallacious to suggest that only the randomized clinical trial can provide valid information or that all information acquired by this technique is valid. Such experimental methods are intended to reduce error and bias and therefore reduce the uncertainty of the result. Uncertainty cannot be eliminated, however. The scientific method is based on increasing probabilities and increasingly refined approximations of truth. Although the randomized clinical trial contributes to these ends, it is neither unique nor perfect. Other techniques may also be useful.

Randomized trials often place physicians in the ethically intolerable position of choosing between the good of the patient and that of society. We urge that such situations be avoided and that other techniques of acquiring clinical information be adopted. . . .

The purpose of the randomized clinical trial is to avoid the problems of observer bias and patient selection. It seems to us that techniques might be developed to deal with these issues in other ways. Randomized clinical trials deal with them in a cumbersome and heavy-handed manner, by requiring large numbers of patients in the hope that random assignment will balance the heterogeneous distribution of patients into the different groups. By observing known characteristics of patients, such as age and sex, and distributing them equally between groups, it is thought that unknown factors important in determining outcomes will also be distributed equally. Surely, other techniques can be developed to deal with both observer bias and patient selection. Prospective studies without randomization, but with the evaluation of patients by uninvolved third parties, should remove observer bias. Prospective matched-pair analysis, in which patients are treated in a manner consistent with their physician's views, ought to help ensure equivalence between the groups and thus mitigate the effect of patient selection, at least with regard to known covariates. With regard to unknown covariates, the security would rest, as in randomized trials, in the enrollment of large numbers of patients and in confirmatory studies. This method would not pose ethical difficulties, since patients would receive the treatment recommended by their physician. They would be included in the study by independent observers matching patients with respect to known characteristics, a process that would not affect patient care and that could be performed independently any number of times.

This brief discussion of alternatives to randomized clinical trials is sketchy and incomplete. We wish only to point out that there may be satisfactory alternatives, not to describe and evaluate them completely. Even if randomized clinical trials were much better than any alternative, however, the ethical dilemmas they present may put their use at variance with the primary obligations of the physician. In this regard, [M.] Angell cautions, "If this commitment to the patient is attenuated, even for so good a cause as benefits to future patients, the implicit assumptions of the doctor-patient relationship are violated." The risk of such attenuation by the randomized trial is great. The AIDS activists have brought this dramatically to the attention of the academic medical community. Techniques appropriate to the laboratory may not be applicable to humans. We must develop and use alternative methods for acquiring clinical knowledge.

Periodical Bibliography

The following articles have been selected to supplement the diverse views presented in this chapter.

Maxine Abrams	"Medical Research Saved My Life," *Good Housekeeping*, November 1991.
George J. Annas and Michael A. Grodin	"Commentary," *Hastings Center Report*, March/April 1991.
Allan Brett	"Ethical Aspects of Human Experimentation in Health Services Research," *JAMA*, April 10, 1991.
Bruce Dobkin	"A Testing Time," *Discover*, May 1990.
Benjamin Freedman, Abraham Fuks, and Charles Weijer	"In Loco Parentis: Minimal Risk as an Ethical Threshold for Research upon Children," *Hastings Center Report*, March/April 1993.
Joan O'C. Hamilton	"Who Told You You Could Sell My Spleen?" *Business Week*, April 23, 1990.
Edmund G. Howe and Edward D. Martin	"Treating the Troops," *Hastings Center Report*, March/April 1991.
Issues	"Considering Experimentation and Elusive Truth: Informed Consent Made Difficult," March/April 1992. Available from SSM Health Care System, 477 N. Lindbergh Blvd., St. Louis, MO 63141.
Laura Weiss Lane, Christine K. Cassel, and Woodward Bennett	"Ethical Aspects of Research Involving Elderly Subjects," *The Journal of Clinical Ethics*, Winter 1990. Available from 107 E. Church St., Frederick, MD 21701.
Karen Lebacqz	"Feminism and Bioethics: An Overview," *Second Opinion*, October 1991. Available from the Park Ridge Center for the Study of Health, Faith, and Ethics, 676 N. St. Clair St., Ste. 450, Chicago, IL 60611.
Carol Levine	"Kids as Guinea Pigs," *Parents*, November 1990.
Pat Roy Mooney	"John Moore's Body," *The New Internationalist*, March 1991.
The Progressive	February 1993. Two articles on the patenting of biological products.
Gary Slutsker	"Patenting Mother Nature," *Forbes*, January 7, 1991.

What Ethics Should Guide Organ Transplants?

Biomedical Ethics

Chapter Preface

In Robin Cook's novel *Coma*, medical student Susan Wheeler is horrified to discover a hospital ward in which patients in a vegetative state are "warehoused," waiting for their organs to be "harvested" for those with money to pay for them. Similar grotesque visions haunt the minds of many who fear that the medical advances that make it possible to save lives by replacing worn-out organs may lead eventually to the dehumanization of the sick and dying, as they become valued not for themselves but for the pieces they can provide for others.

Fueling this fear are the growing skills and knowledge of physicians and researchers who are discovering ever more ways to use fragile and difficult-to-preserve organs, making demand for these organs continue to rise. *Forbes* magazine, for example, reported that in 1990 approximately twenty thousand people were waiting for organs. That number is even higher today. Where are all these organs to come from? Efforts to increase the supply of transplantable organs at present consist primarily of encouraging more voluntary donations. However, other, more extreme practices are occurring as well. For example, in some countries it is common practice for living donors to sell "spare" organs to those who can pay the price. California's Loma Linda Hospital and a few others have experimented with transplanting animal organs into human patients. And Californians Abe and Mary Ayala are one of several couples who have acknowledged conceiving a baby in order to acquire a tissue donor for an ill family member.

While some applaud these efforts to save lives, others fear such practices herald a brave new world in which the lives of some people are considered of little value except as they can contribute to the preservation of the lives of others, who may be richer or more privileged. The authors of the viewpoints in this chapter debate some of the ethical questions that have been raised by the medical advances in organ transplantation.

"In the transplanting of human organs, we have made a start on a road that leads imperceptibly but surely toward a destination that none of us wants to reach."

The Buying and Selling of Organs Raises Serious Ethical Questions

Leon R. Kass

Leon R. Kass is a physician, biochemist, and professor at the University of Chicago. In the following viewpoint, he discusses the moral distaste he feels for organ transplants. His squeamishness, he states, is overcome only by the idea that the gift of an organ by one person can save the life of another. He deeply believes, however, that by "commodifying" organs—making them into commodities that can be bought and sold—humankind will dehumanize itself.

As you read, consider the following questions:

1. Why does Kass find the idea of organ transplants repugnant?
2. In what way does he think organ *donation* is a reaffirmation of the self? Why does he think buying and selling organs, in contrast, is dehumanizing?
3. What is "the destination that none of us wants to reach" that Kass believes the buying and selling of organs will lead to?

From Leon R. Kass, "Organs for Sale?" Reprinted, with permission, from: *The Public Interest*, No. 107 (Spring 1992), pp. 65-86, © 1992 by National Affairs, Inc.

Just in case anyone is expecting to read about new markets for Wurlitzers, let me set you straight. I mean to discuss organ transplantation and, especially, what to think about recent proposals to meet the need for transplantable human organs by permitting or even encouraging their sale and purchase. If the reader will pardon the impropriety, I will not beat around the bush: the subject is human flesh, the goal is the saving of life, the question is, "To market or not to market?"...

Treatment of Corpses

Most of our attitudes regarding invasions of the body and treatment of corpses are carried less by maxims and arguments, more by sentiments and repugnances. They are transmitted inadvertently and indirectly, rarely through formal instruction. For this reason, they are held by some to be suspect, mere sentiments, atavisms tied to superstitions of a bygone age. Some even argue that these repugnances are based mainly on strangeness and unfamiliarity; the strange repels *because* it is unfamiliar. On this view, our squeamishness about dismemberment of corpses is akin to our horror at eating brains or mice. Time and exposure will cure us of these revulsions, especially when there are—as with organ transplantation—such enormous benefits to be won.

These views are, I believe, mistaken. To be sure, as an empirical matter, we can probably get used to many things that once repelled us—organ swapping among them. As Raskolnikov put it, and he should know, "Man gets used to everything—the beast." But I am certain that the repugnances that protect the dignity and integrity of the body are not based solely on strangeness. And they are certainly not irrational. On the contrary, they may just be—like the human body they seek to protect—the very embodiment of reason. Such was the view of Kant, whose title to rationality is second to none, writing in *The Metaphysical Principles of Virtue*:

> To deprive oneself of an integral part or organ (to mutilate oneself), e.g., to *give away* or *sell* a tooth so that it can be planted in the jawbone of another person, or to submit oneself to castration in order to gain an easier livelihood as a singer, and so on, belongs to partial self-murder. But this is not the case with the amputation of a dead organ, or one on the verge of mortification and thus harmful to life. Also, it cannot be reckoned a crime against one's own person to cut off something which is, to be sure, a part, but not an organ of the body, e.g., the hair, although selling one's hair for gain is not entirely free from blame.

Kant, rationalist though he was, understood the rational man's duty to himself as an animal body, precisely because this special animal body was the incarnation of reason:

> [T]o dispose of oneself as a mere means to some end of one's own liking is to degrade the humanity in one's person (*homo noumenon*), which, after all, was entrusted to man (*homo phenomenon*) to preserve.

Man contradicts his rational being by treating his body as a mere means.

Respect for the Living and the Dead

Beginning with notions of propriety, rooted in the meaning of our precarious yet dignified embodiment, we start with a series of presumptions and repugnances *against* treating the human body in the ways that are required for organ transplantation, which really is—once we strip away the trappings of the sterile operating rooms and their astonishing technologies—simply a noble form of cannibalism. Let me summarize these *prima facie* points of departure.

• Regarding *living donors*, there is a presumption against self-mutilation, even when good can come of it, a presumption, by the way, widely endorsed in the practice of medicine: Following venerable principles of medical ethics, surgeons are loath to cut into a healthy body not for its own benefit. As a result, most of them will not perform transplants using kidneys or livers from unrelated living donors.

• Regarding *cadaver donation*, there is a *beginning* presumption that mutilating a corpse defiles its integrity, that utilization of its parts violates its dignity, that ceremonial disposition of the total remains is the fitting way to honor and respect the life that once this body lived. Further, because of our body's inherent connection with the embodied lives of parents, spouses, and children, the common law properly mandates the body of the deceased to next of kin, in order to perform last rites, to mourn together in the presence of the remains, to say ceremonial farewell, and to mark simultaneously the connection to and the final separation from familial flesh. The deep wisdom of these sentiments and ways explains why it is a strange and indeed upsetting departure to allow the will of the deceased to determine the disposition of his remains and to direct the donation of his organs after death: for these very bodily remains are proof of the limits of his will and the fragility of his life, after which they "belong" properly to the family for the reasons and purposes just indicated. These reflections also explain why doctors—who know better than philosophers and economists the embodied nature of all personal life—are, despite their interest in organ transplantation, so reluctant to press the next of kin for permission to remove organs. This, and not fear of lawsuit, is the reason why doctors will not harvest organs without the family's consent, even in cases in which the deceased was a known, card-carrying organ donor.

• Regarding the *recipients of transplantation*, there is some primordial revulsion over confusion of personal identity, implicit in the thought of walking around with someone else's liver or heart. To be sure, for most recipients life with mixed identity is vastly preferable to the alternative, and the trade is easily accepted. Also, the alien additions are tucked safety inside, hidden from sight. Yet transplantation as such—especially of vital organs—troubles the easygoing presumption of self-in-body, and ceases to do so only if one comes to accept a strict person-body dualism or adopts, against the testimony of one's own lived experience, the proposition that a person is or lives only in his brain-and-or-mind. Even the silent body speaks up to oppose transplantation, in the name of integrity, selfhood, and identity: its immune system, which protects the body against all foreign intruders, naturally rejects tissues and organs transplanted from another body.

• Finally, regarding *privacy and publicity*, though we may celebrate the life-saving potential of transplantation or even ordinary surgery, we are rightly repelled by the voyeurism of the media, and the ceaseless chatter about this person's donation and that person's new heart. We have good reason to deplore the coarsening of sensibilities that a generation ago thought it crude of Lyndon Johnson to show off his surgical scar, but that now is quite comfortable with television in the operating suite, request for organ donation in the newspaper, talk-show confessions of conceiving children to donate bone marrow, and the generalized talk of spare parts and pressed flesh.

The Burden of Proof

I have, I am aware, laid it on thick. But I believe it is necessary to do so. For we cannot begin in the middle, taking organ transplantation simply for granted. We must see that, from the point of view of decency and seemliness and propriety, there are scruples to be overcome and that organ transplantation must bear the burden of proof. I confess that, on balance, I believe the burden can be easily shouldered, for the saving of life is indeed a great good acknowledged by all. Desiring the end, we will the means, and reason thus helps us overcome our repugnances—and, unfortunately, leads us to forget what this costs us, in coin of shame and propriety. We are able to overcome the restraints against violating the integrity of dead bodies; less easily, but easily enough for kin, we overcome our scruple against self-mutilation in allowing and endorsing living donation—though here we remain especially sensitive to the dangers of coercion and manipulation of family ties.

How have we been able to do so? Primarily by insisting on the principle not only of voluntary consent but also of *free donation*. We have avoided the simple utilitarian calculation and not pursued the policy that would get us the most organs. We have, in short, acknowledged the weight of the non-utilitarian considerations, of the concerns of propriety. Indeed, to legitimate the separation of organs from bodies, we have insisted on a principle which obscures or even, in a sense, denies the fact of ultimate separation. For in a *gift* of an organ—by its living "owner"—as with any gift, what is given is not merely the physical entity. Like any gift, a *donated* organ carries with it the donor's generous good will. It is accompanied, so to speak, by the generosity of soul of the donor. Symbolically, the "aliveness" of the organ requisite for successful transplant bespeaks also the expansive liveliness of the donor—even, or especially, after his death. Thus organ removal, the partial alienation-of-self-from-body, turns out to be, in this curious way, a *reaffirmation* of the self's embodiment, thanks to the generous act of donation.

We are now ready to think about buying and selling, and questions regarding the body as property.

Property

The most common objections to permitting the sale of body parts, especially from live donors, have to do with matters of equity, exploitation of the poor and the unemployed and the dangers of abuse—not excluding theft and even murder to obtain valuable commodities. People deplore the degrading sale, a sale made in desperation, especially when the seller is selling something so precious as a part of his own body. Others deplore the rich man's purchase, and would group life-giving organs with other most basic goods that should not be available to the rich when the poor can't afford them (like allowing people to purchase substitutes for themselves in the military draft). Lloyd Cohen's proposal for a futures market in organs was precisely intended to avoid these evils: through it he addresses only increasing the supply without embracing a market for allocation—thus avoiding special privileges for the rich, and by buying early from the living but harvesting only from the dead he believes—I think mistakenly—that we escape the danger of exploiting the poor. (This and other half-market proposals seeking to protect the poor from exploitation would in fact cheat them out of what their organs would fetch, were the rich compelled to bid and buy in a truly open market.) . . .

Torn between sympathy and disgust, some observers would have it both ways: they would permit sale, but ban advertising and criminalize brokering (i.e., legalize prostitutes, prosecute pimps), presumably to eliminate coercive pressure from unscrupulous middlemen. But none of these analysts, it seems to me, has faced the question squarely. For if there were nothing fundamentally wrong with trading organs in the first place, why should it bother us that some people will make their living at it? The objection in the name of exploitation and inequity—however important for determining policy—seems to betray deeper objections, unacknowledged, to the thing itself—objections of the sort I dealt with in the discussion of propriety. For it is difficult to understand why someone who sees absolutely no difficulty at all with transplantation and donation should have such trouble sanctioning sale. . . .

Let us put aside questions about property and free contract, and think only about buying and selling. Never mind our rights, what would it mean to fully commercialize the human body even, say, under state monopoly? What, regardless of political system, is the moral and philosophical difference between giving an organ and selling it, or between receiving it as a gift and buying it?

Commodification

The idea of commodification of human flesh repels us, quite properly I would say, because we sense that the human body especially belongs in that category of things that defy or resist commensuration—like love or friendship or life itself. To claim that these things are "priceless" is not to insist that they are of infinite worth or that one cannot calculate (albeit very roughly, and then only with aid of very crude simplifying assumptions) how much it costs to sustain or support them. Rather it is to claim that the bulk of their meaning and their human worth do not lend themselves to quantitative measure; for this reason, we hold them to be incommensurable, not only morally but factually.

Against this view, it can surely be argued that the entire system of market exchange rests on our arbitrary but successful attempts to commensurate the (factually) incommensurable. The genius of money is precisely that it solves by convention the problem of natural incommensurability, say between oranges and widgets, or between manual labor and the thinking time of economists. The possibility of civilization altogether rests on this conventional means of exchange, as the ancient Greeks noted by deriving the name for money, *nomisma*, from the root *nomos* meaning "convention"—that which has been settled by human agreement—and showing how this fundamental convention made possible commerce, leisure, and the establishment of gentler views of justice.

Yet the purpose of instituting such a conventional measure was to facilitate the satisfaction of *natural* human needs and the desires for well-being and, eventually, to encourage the full flowering of human possibility. Some notion of need or perceived human good provided always the latent non-conventional standard behind the nomismatic convention—tacitly, to be sure. And there's the rub: In due course, the standard behind money, being hidden, eventually becomes forgotten, and the counters of worth become taken for worth itself.

Truth to tell, commodification by conventional commensuration always risks the homogenization of worth, and even the homogenization of things, all under the aspect of quantity. In many transactions, we do not mind or suffer or even notice. Yet the human soul finally rebels against the principle, whenever it strikes closest to home. Consider, for example, why there is such widespread dislike of the pawnbroker. It is not only that he profits from our misfortunes and sees the shame of our having to part with heirlooms and other items said (inadequately) to have "sentimental value." It is especially because he will not and cannot appreciate their human and personal worth and pays us only their market price. How much more will we object to those who would commodify our very being?

We surpass all defensible limits of such conventional commodification when we contemplate making the convention-maker—the human being—just another one of the commensurables. The end comes to be treated as mere means. Selling our bodies, we come perilously close to selling out our souls. There is even a danger in contemplating such a prospect—for if we come to think about ourselves like pork bellies, pork bellies we will become.

Manipulating the Human Body

We have, with some reluctance, overcome our repugnance at the exploitative manipulation of one human body to serve the life and health of another. We have managed to justify our present arrangements not only on grounds of utility or freedom but also and especially on the basis of generosity, in which the generous deed of the giver is inseparable from the organ given. To allow the commodification of these exchanges is to forget altogether the impropriety overcome in allowing donation and transplantation in the first place. And it is to turn generosity into trade, gratitude into compensation. It is to treat the most delicate of human affairs as if everything is reducible to its price.

There is a euphemism making the rounds in these discussions that makes my point. Eager to encourage more donation, but loath to condone or to speak about buying and selling organs, some have called for the practice of "rewarded gifting"—in which the donor is rewarded for his generosity, not paid for his organ. Some will smile at what looks like double-talk or hypocrisy, but even if it is hypocrisy, it is thereby a tribute paid to virtue. Rewards are given for good deeds, whereas fees are charged for services, and prices are paid merely for goods. If we must continue to practice organ transplantation, let us do so on good behavior.

Freely Giving Organs

Anticipating the problem we now face, Paul Ramsey twenty years ago proposed that we copy for organ donation a practice sometimes used in obtaining blood: those who freely give can, when in need, freely receive. "Families that shared in premortem giving of organs could share in freely receiving if one of them needs transplant therapy. This would be—if workable—a civilizing exchange of benefit that is not the same as commerce in organs." Ramsey saw in this possibility of organized generosity a way to promote civilized community and to make virtue grow out of dire necessity. These, too, are precious "commodities," and provide an additional reason for believing that the human body and the extraordinary generosity in the gift of its parts are altogether too precious to be commodified.

Losing Respect for the Dead

There is, no doubt, a big demand for organs for transplantation, but, to an old fellow like me, it all has an unsavory feeling about it: you are taking from cadavers or from living human beings, organs they are prepared to get rid of, or, as is tragically the case, from people in the world who are so poor, so without the necessities of life, that they are prepared to offer their own organs for sale in order to be able to satisfy themselves in other directions. Now to me, at any rate, this is a sort of very sad thing. One cannot actually nail down why it seems horrible that a kidney should be sold for a large sum of money, or that there are people so desperately in need of kidneys that they are prepared to pay very large sums of money for them, but to me these contracts have something very creepy and unpleasant about them. . . . The cadaver has come to have a market value, leaving no place for requiems, prayers, or mourning with kidneys, hearts, eyeballs and other such items up for sale.

Malcolm Muggeridge, *Human Life Review*, Spring 1992.

The arguments I have offered are not easy to make. I am all too well aware that they can be countered, that their appeal is largely to certain hard-to-articulate intuitions and sensibilities that I at least believe belong intimately to the human experience of our own humanity. Precious though they might be, they do not exhaust the human picture, far from it. And perhaps, in the present case, they should give way to rational calculation, market mechanisms, and even naked commodification of human flesh—all in the service of saving life at lowest cost (though, parenthetically, it would be worth a whole separate discussion to consider whether, in the longer view, there are not cheaper, more effective, and less indecent means to save lives, say, through preventive measures that forestall end-stage renal disease now requiring transplantation: the definition of both need and efficiency are highly contingent, and we should beware of allowing them to be defined for us by those technologists—like transplant surgeons—wedded to present practice). Perhaps this is not the right place to draw a line or to make a stand.

Consider, then, a slightly more progressive and enterprising proposal, one anticipated by my colleague, Willard Gaylin, in an essay, "Harvesting the Dead," written in 1974. Mindful of all the possible uses of newly dead—or perhaps not-quite-dead-bodies, kept in their borderline condition by continuous artificial respiration and assisted circulation, intact, warm, pink, recognizably you or me, but brain dead. Gaylin imagines the multiple medically beneficial uses to which the bioemporium of such "neomorts" could be put: the neomorts could, for example, allow physicians-in-training to practice pelvic examinations and tracheal intubations without shame or fear of doing damage; they could serve as unharmable subjects for medical experimentation and drug testing, provide indefinite supplies of blood, marrow, and skin, serve as factories to manufacture hormones and antibodies, or, eventually, be dismembered for transplantable spare parts. Since the newly dead body really is a precious resource, why not really put it to full and limitless use?

Body Farming

Gaylin's scenario is not so far-fetched. Proposals to undertake precisely such body-farming have been seriously discussed among medical scientists in private. The technology for maintaining neomorts is already available. Indeed, in the past few years, a publicly traded corporation has opened a national chain of large, specialized nursing homes—or should we rather call them nurseries?—for the care and feeding solely of persons in persistent vegetative state or ventilator-dependent irreversible coma. Roughly ten establishments, each housing several hundred of such beings, already exist. All that would be required to turn them into Gaylin's bioemporia would be a slight revision in the definition of death (already proposed for other reasons)—to shift from death of the whole brain to death of the cortex and the higher centers—plus the will not to let these valuable resources go to waste. (The company's stock, by the way, has more than quadrupled; perhaps someone is already preparing

71

plans for mergers and manufacture.)

Repulsive? You bet. Useful? Without doubt. Shall we go forward into this brave new world?

Forward we are going, without anyone even asking the question. In the twenty-five years since I began thinking about these matters, our society has overcome longstanding taboos and repugnances to accept test-tube fertilization, commercial sperm-banking, surrogate motherhood, abortion on demand, exploitation of fetal tissue, patenting of living human tissue, gender-change surgery, liposuction and body shops, the widespread shuttling of human parts, assisted-suicide practiced by doctors, and the deliberate generation of human beings to serve as transplant donors—not to speak about massive changes in the culture regarding shame, privacy, and exposure. Perhaps more worrisome than the changes themselves is the coarsening of sensibilities and attitudes, and the irreversible effects on our imaginations and the way we come to conceive of ourselves. For there is a sad irony in our biomedical project, accurately anticipated in Aldous Huxley's *Brave New World*: We expend enormous energy and vast sums of money to preserve and prolong bodily life, but in the process our embodied life is stripped of its gravity and much of its dignity. This is, in a word, progress as tragedy.

In the transplanting of human organs, we have made a start on a road that leads imperceptibly but surely toward a destination that none of us wants to reach. A divination of this fact produced reluctance at the start. Yet the first step, overcoming reluctance, was defensible on benevolent and rational grounds: save life using organs no longer useful to their owners and otherwise lost to worms.

Now, embarked on the journey, we cannot go back. Yet we are increasingly troubled by the growing awareness that there is neither a natural nor a rational place to stop. Precedent justifies extension, so does rational calculation: We are in a warm bath that warms up so imperceptibly that we don't know when to scream.

And this is perhaps the most interesting and the most tragic element of my dilemma—and it is not my dilemma alone. I don't want to encourage: yet I cannot simply condemn. I refuse to approve, yet I cannot moralize. How, in this matter of organs for sale, as in so much of modern life, is one to conduct one's thoughts if one wishes neither to be a crank nor to yield what is best in human life to rational analysis and the triumph of technique? Is poor reason impotent to do anything more than to recognize and state this tragic dilemma?

"The current system, relying as it does
exclusively on altruism, is unable to end the
[organ] shortage."

The Buying and Selling of
Organs Saves Lives

Ronald Bailey

Many of the people waiting for organ transplants never receive
them. In the following viewpoint, Ronald Bailey discusses the
lack of available organs and concludes that one way to increase
their availability is to allow them to be bought and sold as other
commodities are. Bailey points out that blood and plasma are already bought and sold. Money for organs, he states, will provide
the motivation that pure altruism has not.

As you read, consider the following questions:

1. Why, according to Bailey, have required consent laws, which
   mandate that hospitals ask families to donate the organs of
   their dying relatives, failed to increase the number of organs
   available for transplants?
2. What forms of compensation other than "cold cash" does the
   author suggest might be used?
3. According to Bailey, how does organ availability in the United
   States compare to that in other countries?

Ronald Bailey, "Should I Be Allowed to Buy Your Kidney?" *Forbes*, May 28, 1990. Reprinted
by permission of *Forbes* magazine, © Forbes, Inc., 1990.

Randy Creech, a 43-year-old executive with an Exxon subsidiary in Houston, has needed a new heart since a viral infection all but destroyed his heart muscle. Creech, the father of two, has been on the Texas Heart Institute's transplant waiting list for three months. He works part time, all the while waiting for a pager at his side to beep, signaling that he has four hours to get to the hospital where surgeons will be waiting with a fresh heart. There are 20 people of his blood type on a list of 60.

Modern medicine has worked miracles for people who need a new heart or kidney or other organs. Demand for organ transplants has increased sharply. Unfortunately, there are no miracles on the supply side. Thousands of would-be recipients die every year while waiting.

Can anything be done to increase the supply of transplant organs? Some doctors are very quietly talking about compensating donors.

That's right: I'll pay you $5,000 for one of your kidneys. Not enough? How about $20,000?

Organ Trafficking

Right now trafficking in organs is punishable by big fines and imprisonment in the U.S. and throughout much of the industrialized world—although commercial transactions in blood are not. But not every country observes the taboo. Circumstantial evidence is accumulating that the Republic of China has turned the transplant business into a source of hard currency. The government, which reportedly has executed 11,000 people in the past decade, prefers using a shot through the head. By so doing, the executioners maximize doctors' chances of retrieving useful organs from the prisoner's body. "Execution by organ donation" is how the ghoulish process is described by Brian Broznick, executive director of the Pittsburgh Organ Transplant Foundation, the U.S.' largest organ procurement organization. The Chinese Embassy in Washington denies that organs are taken from executed prisoners and used for transplantation.

True or not, it is a fact that well-to-do Singaporeans and Hong Kong citizens have traveled to China for transplanted organs, in most cases kidneys.

However distasteful this may sound, a strong case can be made that people should be allowed to sell and buy human organs. The supply continues to fall short of demand. After a period of growth in the early 1980s, the number of donations has leveled off.

In an effort to bolster faltering voluntary donations, Congress passed a law in 1988 requiring hospitals to ask families for permission to donate the organs from their recently deceased family members. Sadly, the law has produced gruesome sessions in which the doctor first breaks the bad news about Uncle Isador, then asks for his organs. "Required request laws are a joke," says Broznick, the Pittsburgh organ executive.

There are some bright spots. A Boston consulting firm, Corporate Decisions, Inc., is working with the regional Kentucky organ procurement organization. The program focuses on hospitals that treat serious head injuries and trains hospital employees in how to deal with the emotional distress of donor families. The consultants sensibly recommend that the request for organ donation come at a time after the family has been informed of the death. The experimental program has helped increase organ donations by 20%—a significant step in the right direction.

But it is by no means certain that voluntary donations will ever provide sufficient supply, given advancements in medical science and in organ transplanting. "I can't see why the only persons not to make a legitimate degree of financial advantage from transplantation are the people who give the organs," says Dr. John Dossetor, a nephrologist (kidney doctor) and a bioethicist in Edmonton, Alberta. "Everybody else is living by it, including myself."

There are any number of ways to compensate donors or their families. The compensation can come in the form of straight cash, or coverage of burial expenses, or through estate tax breaks or college education benefits for survivors.

When people think of organ donations, they usually think of cadaver donations—organs removed from dead bodies. But there is another possibility: live donors. There were 1,822 such donors of kidneys in 1989 in the U.S. Increasingly, there are more live donations of bone marrow and pieces of liver; like blood, liver can regenerate to produce whole organs in both donor and recipient.

Living Donors

In the world's poorer countries, hospitals rarely have the equipment or trained staff to save organs for transplant. Nor can most of these countries afford hemodialysis facilities, thus, in effect, sentencing patients with kidney failure to certain death. In the case of kidney failure, the only real solution in many poor countries is to buy a kidney from a living donor, in a straightforward commercial transaction.

Consider the case of A.S. Reddy, a 45-year-old corporate secretary at the publishing house Orient-Longman in Hyderabad, India. His kidneys failed in 1987. None of his siblings was an appropriate donor. Reddy was fortunate to be able to afford private renal dialysis while his doctor, K.C. Reddy (no relation), looked for an appropriate donor. After just three months on dialysis, Reddy was successfully implanted with a kidney from Mrs. Velangani Vitalravi, a 25-year-old garment factory worker and mother of two.

"I had no choice but to pay for a kidney," the recipient says. Surgeon K. C. Reddy phrases his ethical response in this way: "Either I buy, or they die."

How Much Are You Worth?

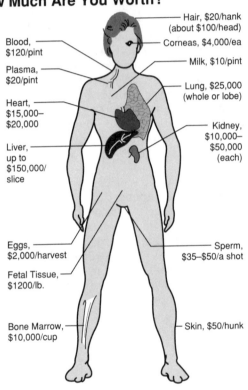

Dead Whole Body

$50,000 if dead less than 15 hours

$1,000 if dead more than 15 hours

Alive Whole Body

Guinea Pigging: $100 per day plus room & board

Working: $4.25 per hour, minimum wage

Blood, $120/pint

Plasma, $20/pint

Heart, $15,000–$20,000

Liver, up to $150,000/slice

Eggs, $2,000/harvest

Fetal Tissue, $1200/lb.

Bone Marrow, $10,000/cup

Hair, $20/hank (about $100/head)

Corneas, $4,000/ea

Milk, $10/pint

Lung, $25,000 (whole or lobe)

Kidney, $10,000–$50,000 (each)

Sperm, $35–$50/a shot

Skin, $50/hunk

Source: *Sell Yourself to Science* by Jim Hogshire.

What about the lady who parted with one of her two kidneys? Mrs. Vitalravi used her money to buy a piece of land in her home town of Ambattur, just outside Madras, where she plans to build a house one day. Her husband also sold one of his kidneys and used the money to pay off debts and cover his sister's dowry and wedding costs.

Dr. Reddy, who did the operation, was trained in Madras, spent a year at Sinai Hospital in Baltimore, worked for five years in hospitals in England and ultimately returned to India in the early 1980s. His transplant team has performed more than 600 transplants to date—all of which involved kidneys obtained from living donors, 450 of whom were unrelated. Reddy's clinic also handles the financial arrangements, in order to exclude middlemen who might coerce or blackmail donors to sell a kidney.

A complete operation in Dr. Reddy's clinic, including hospital costs, testing and donated organ, costs $5,000 for an Indian recipient, or $8,000 for a foreigner. (In the U.S. a kidney transplant operation typically costs $51,000 and is covered by Medicare.) Reddy pays kidney donors $1,800—about six times the average annual wage in India.

Human Capital

Thus are organs literally human capital. According to Reddy, one kidney donor bought a small farm, another set up shop as a shoemaker, a third set up a poultry business. Will Americans seek kidney transplants in India and other places where the organs are available if the supply bottleneck gets much worse?

"I have no doubt that it will occur," says Dallas nephrologist Alan Hull. "As the waiting list grows, I have to say to patients, 'Look, you have a rare blood type and you're a high reactor. The waiting time for you will be five to ten years, which is longer than your life expectancy, so while I'd love to give you a transplant, I don't think I can offer it to you.' If that person has money and there's a kidney in Bombay—their chances are just under 50-50, let's say—you know what will happen. They're going to buy one."

Adds Hull: "When you bring that scenario up at medical society meetings, no one wants to talk about it."

Under current U.S. law, a living donor cannot be paid for his or her organ, but can specify who is to receive it. That simply means that most live kidney donors are related to the recipients. Yet doctors will tell you that illegal compensation is sometimes exchanged.

"The fact is that many [living donors] are getting compensated under the table," says Dr. Hull of Dallas. "Suddenly a [donor] gets a new business, or a new house or a new car, just after he's donated to his nephew or some friend. And medicine has trouble with that, because we don't want to know about it." Dr. James Light of Washington, D.C.-based Washington Hospital Center, one of the largest transplant centers in the nation, estimates that in perhaps 15% to 20% of the cases between living related donors, some economic benefit is exchanged.

It's one of the toughest ethical questions in medicine: Doctors want more organ donations, but they don't want to see kidneys bought and sold like cars or sides of beef.

"I would look for ways of legalizing organ sales, and knowing all that I know about our society, I'd do it with oversight and regulation, so that nobody would worry about it," says H. Tristam Engelhardt Jr., a bioethicist and physician at Baylor College of Medicine in Houston.

Paying for Organs

Current law says that no money can change hands for an organ. Most living donors give to a blood relative, where the chances are greatest of a good match. Occasionally, however, people who are not blood related—spouses, friends, lovers—are capable of donating. But before they can, doctors want to satisfy themselves that the donor's motive is purely altruistic. Dr. Ronald Ferguson, a nephrologist at Ohio State University, says he looks for "some sort of emotional tie to make sure that the kidney is given in the right spirit."

The whole issue is so wrapped in emotion that it is difficult to get even rational discussion. When Congress passed the National Organ Transplant Act in 1984, it made the buying and selling of organs an illegal act punishable by fines of up to $50,000 or five years in prison, or both. Reports of foreigners buying their way to the top of U.S. transplant lists helped mobilize support for the legislation and won a 1986 Pulitzer Prize for the *Pittsburgh Press.*

In Britain recently, Dr. Maurice Bewick, a prominent kidney transplant surgeon, was suspended from private practice for two years by the General Medical Council after he transplanted a kidney into a Turkish man. The patient had paid $4,000 to the donor, another Turk, who had accompanied the man on a trip to London for the operation. At the time of the operation, the transaction was not illegal in Britain, although the British Transplantation Society's guidelines forbade such deals. A colleague also lost his license. Soon after the case arose in January 1989, the British Parliament outlawed the purchase of organs for transplantation.

At the root of the fundamental questions posed by transplants are the great leaps forward in the area of drugs that reduce the chances that the recipient's body will reject a donated organ. Thus donors and recipients need not worry so much about matching anymore.

During rejection, the human immune system tries to destroy transplanted organs as though they were invading disease organisms. Two powerful new immunosuppressant drugs not yet on the market are Syntex Corp.'s RS 61443, and FK 506, developed by Japan's Fujisawa Pharmaceutical. FK 506 is 50 to 100 times more potent in controlling transplant tissue rejection than Sandoz Ltd.'s cyclosporine, the immunosuppressant whose approval in 1983 ushered in the modern era of transplantation.

Transplant patients must take immunosuppressant drugs like

cyclosporine for the rest of their lives. A year's supply of cyclosporine A costs between $3,000 and $7,000. Eventually, the experimental drugs are expected both to lower the cost of cyclosporine and to increase further the likelihood of a transplant's success.

Technology is enabling doctors to keep organs longer outside the human body. A new preservation solution, Viaspan, developed by Dr. Folkert Belzer and James Southard at the University of Wisconsin and now marketed by Du Pont, will let a donated organ be shipped safely for longer distances than ever before. Previously livers could be preserved for only 8 hours; now they can be preserved for up to 32 hours. Clinical trials indicate that hearts can be preserved 12 hours instead of 4. And with kidneys, Viaspan has shown a 30% reduction in the need for dialysis after a transplant. . . .

Why is it perfectly legal to sell so-called soft tissues like blood and semen in the U.S., but illegal to sell fetal tissue, bone marrow, corneas or solid organs outright for transplant?

As is usual with difficult moral questions, decision making is passing by default to the courts. In 1988 the California Court of Appeals ruled that a patient has a property interest in his cells. It did not rule on whether the patient was entitled to compensation and it refrained from legalizing free trade in body parts.

Selling Body Parts Is Ethical

There is nothing immoral about renting or selling your body. The idea that there is something wrong with this is rooted in the same tradition as the fantasy that "if you work hard enough someday the boss will notice you and promote you." In other words, it serves the purposes of those folks who have no problem with breaking your back all your life then, when you are dead, mining your corpse for life-saving organs. On the contrary, one can make a very good case that *refusing* to allow people to sell the most personal of all property is immoral, resulting in the waste of valuable resources and the loss of life.

Jim Hogshire, *Sell Yourself to Science*, 1992.

The patient, John Moore, had his malignant spleen removed. His physician at the University of California at Los Angeles found that cells from his spleen produced a protein that was effective in fighting a kind of leukemia. Moore asserted that the doctor profited by selling a cell line cultured from Moore's cells to Genetics Institute, a Boston biotech firm, and its partner, Sandoz. Genetics Institute appealed the appeals court ruling. A hearing was held before the California Supreme Court, and the case is still pending.

Should transplantable hearts, kidneys, bone marrow and other organs be treated by the law similarly to the way blood is treated? Despite the extraordinary success of the Red Cross in producing voluntary blood donations, it is easy to forget that there is still a successful—and safe—commercial plasma industry in this country. Plasma is also a source of export income. The U.S. supplies 60% of the world's $2-billion-per-year plasma market. Countries relying solely on voluntary blood collections, such as Britain and Japan, must import commercial American plasma in order to overcome their shortages.

Altruism Not Enough

Increasing the supply of blood plasma through a combination of voluntary and commercial means may point the way for increasing the supply of transplant organs. The current system, relying as it does exclusively on altruism, is unable to end the shortage. It is time for the transplantation community, policymakers and the public at large to consider seriously proposals that will invest private property rights in cadaver donors' families and, in the case of bone marrow and perhaps livers and kidneys, in the donors themselves.

Dr. J. Wesley Alexander, a transplant surgeon who chairs the United Network for Organ Sharing donations committee, says, "I think that when push comes to shove, the public has to make a decision as to whether they would rather see people die on dialysis while leading a fairly unsatisfactory life . . . or to allow the buying and selling of human organs." It is an excruciatingly difficult decision, like most thrown up by modern medicine's miracle workers.

"The government has for too long resisted establishing and funding a national policy to encourage an adequate supply . . . of donated organs and tissues."

More Organs for Transplants Must Be Found

Joel L. Swerdlow and Fred H. Cate

As more organs become transplantable, the demand for them grows. Authors Joel L. Swerdlow and Fred H. Cate report that in 1989, nearly seventeen hundred people were saved by heart transplants, but another sixteen hundred did not receive the heart they needed. More than eleven thousand people received other types of transplants. But again, far more people did not receive needed organs. In the following viewpoint, Swerdlow and Cate ask what can be done to increase the supply of transplantable organs. One solution, they suggest, is an efficient national organ registry.

As you read, consider the following questions:

1. According to Swerdlow and Cate, how many people die each year whose organs could be harvested for use by others but are not?
2. The authors cite several impediments to increasing the transplantable organ supply. Name three.
3. What problems do the authors feel would be solved by an efficient national organ registry?

Joel L. Swerdlow and Fred H. Cate, "Why Transplants Don't Happen," *The Atlantic*, October 1990. Reprinted with permission.

In 1989 organ transplants saved or dramatically improved the lives of more than 13,000 Americans. Heart transplants alone saved 1,673 lives. But 1,600 people continue to wait for new hearts; almost a third of them have waited longer than six months. A third will die before they receive a heart. The situation is similar for other organs (kidneys, lungs, livers, pancreases) and tissues (bone, skin, corneas, ligaments, tendons, blood vessels, heart valves). Surgeons performed 8,886 kidney transplants in the United States in 1989. But more than 17,000 people continue to wait for kidneys. Thousands of patients face near-certain death unless they receive bone-marrow transplants. All the while, there are people living in America who could donate small amounts of their marrow and save them. These potential donors are never contacted, because no one knows who they are. Every year tens of thousands of life-enhancing or life-giving operations cannot be performed for lack of organs and tissues, and shortages of organs and tissues stymie research projects to fight fatal diseases.

These shortages need not exist. Almost 2.2 million people die every year in the United States. As many as 25,000 of those people would qualify medically as organ donors; fewer than 4,000 actually donate. The same shortage applies to tissues, which are used increasingly to restore sight and hearing, save cancerous limbs from amputation, and treat burn victims. Many of those 2.2 million people could donate valuable tissues; fewer than 45,000 people do so. According to Raymond Pollak, a transplant surgeon at the University of Illinois in Chicago, transplantation confronts a "shortage in the face of plenty."

Why the Shortage?

A number of factors lie behind this dramatic and deadly shortfall. Even many of those in favor of the donation of organs and tissues find discussing their own death or that of a loved one difficult; often people simply fail to act on their desire to help others. Present law exacerbates the tendency to procrastinate by assuming that any given person wishes *not* to donate organs or tissues upon death, unless that person has indicated otherwise. A person may, for example, sign a donor card. Doctors and hospitals, however, fear professional criticism and lawsuits if they procure organs against the wishes of the next of kin, even if the deceased has indicated a desire to be a donor. A donor card is therefore useless unless the next of kin approve the donation. Under laws enacted in every state and the District of Columbia, a spouse or parent or adult child can approve the donation of a decedent's organs and tissues. But too few people discuss donation with their relatives, and following the death of a loved one the grieving next of kin rarely have donation on their minds.

Many health-care workers often fail even to raise the possibility of donation with the next of kin, despite laws and regulations requiring them to do so.

The law also poses an obstacle by not clarifying who "owns" a donated organ or tissue. The California Supreme Court further confused the issue when it ruled, in *Moore v. Regents of the University of California*, that whatever property interests John Moore at one time possessed in his spleen, there were "several reasons to doubt" whether he retained any ownership interest following its removal during surgery. The court held that on the other hand, if Moore's physicians failed to inform Moore that they were likely to profit from the use of tissue taken from his spleen, then they may have violated their professional obligations to their patient. (Cells from the spleen were used to produce the drug interferon and other lucrative products.) The *Moore* decision is not binding outside California. Moreover, it is not clear that the case relates to the ownership of organs and tissues donated after death, and no other court has yet addressed this issue.

Organs as Property

Some scholars suggest that if officials treated human organs and tissues with the same respect they accord to real property, such as a television or a house (which the legal system acts immediately and forcefully to protect upon the death of the owner), a far greater supply of transplantable body parts would result. The state and the next of kin would respect the decedent's wish to donate organs and tissues, just as they respect the decedent's wishes regarding the disposition of other property. If the decedent had not communicated any decision about donation, the next of kin would be forced to confront the issue— along with issues about the disposition of the rest of the estate— and might better appreciate the value of organs and tissues.

Because there is no automatic transferral of property interests in organs and tissues upon death to patients on the waiting list, no one watches out for the interests of would-be recipients. And the fact that people die every day because our health-care system discards lifesaving organs arouses no comment.

A legal determination by Congress or the courts as to who owns donated organs and tissues—the potential recipient, the procurement organization, or a national network linking transplant centers—would help assure that the law protected those it now largely ignores.

Obtaining consent is only the first of the problems facing transplantation. Once consent is obtained, the organ or tissue must be removed, a recipient must be identified, the body part must be transported to that recipient (or, in some cases, processed for storage, which may last several years), and then it must be transplanted.

But the systems needed to provide rapid and efficient coordination are lacking. For instance, a federally funded computerized national registry and a variety of private registries compete to identify bone-marrow donors, who, like blood donors, are living. Patients in need of a transplant must pay to search the national registry, yet they may still miss the name of a potentially lifesaving donor who happens to be listed on a different registry. A young woman in Denver recently mangled her arm in an automobile accident. An elbow taken from a cadaver and stored in a local bone bank made her whole again. Her surgeon told reporters that she was "lucky" that a bone her size had been available in Denver. Why did she have to rely on luck? A resident of Denver can get airplane or hotel reservations anywhere in the world in a matter of minutes. Physicians should be able to order a bone by computer from any city in the country.

Today different coordination mechanisms exist for organs and for tissues; different coordination mechanisms also exist for transplants and for body parts for research. All these systems have their problems, and cooperation among them is almost nonexistent.

The most elaborate system for coordinating supply and demand for organs is the Organ Procurement and Transplantation Network, which connects fifty-two organ-procurement organizations and 250 transplant centers twenty-four hours a day. This network is the result of a 1984 compromise between proponents of government coordination and Reagan Administration opponents of any federal involvement all. As a result of the compromise, the transplant network enjoys a monopoly on coordination—but with respect only to organs, not to tissues or body parts for research. Even for this limited task the network is significantly underfunded. Its total annual budget, by law, may not exceed $2 million; the largest annual appropriation it has ever received was $1.5 million. Compared with other federally funded data bases—not to mention private networks for airline reservations and auto parts—this money is insignificant.

Organ Procurement

Some critics charge that the operator of the Organ Procurement and Transplantation Network—the United Network for Organ Sharing (UNOS), in Richmond, Virginia—does not run the network efficiently. Despite its statutory monopoly on information relating to organs available for transplant and people waiting for organs, UNOS has yet to provide patients, the public, and the medical profession with important data that would show differences in age, sex, race, and severity of illness among patients at all of the transplant centers.

More significant, critics have charged that UNOS has greatly exceeded its original statutory mandate and made fundamental policy decisions about who should have access to organs. For instance, UNOS has promulgated guidelines on how to weigh various criteria—such as length of time on the waiting list, medical necessity, and the location of the donated organ relative to that of the potential recipient—in determining who on the waiting list will have a chance to live and who will almost certainly die. Until recently federal law required that all transplant centers and organ-procurement organizations abide by those rules, even though UNOS is a private organization. A decision by the Department of Health and Human Services, however, now subjects UNOS rules to the department's approval.

James F. Blumstein, a professor at Vanderbilt University Law School, has observed that UNOS's evolution from a voluntary network into a "comprehensive, top-down, coercive" system runs counter to the trend in favor of competition and decentralization in other facets of health-care policy. Congress must decide whether to condone this development or to permit competition in organ procurement and supply. If Congress chooses in favor of centralization, it must determine whether to permit UNOS to engage in activities other than operating the network and whether to expand its mandate to include tissues and body parts for research. Congress will also have to consider how to ensure that the network has the resources necessary to fulfill its responsibilities.

The area of greatest growth in transplantation is not organs but tissues. A healthy donor can provide at least thirty kinds of tissue, many of which can be taken from the body fifteen or more hours after death. But without an equivalent, for tissue, of the Organ Procurement and Transplantation Network, half a dozen overlapping private national networks have emerged. Many tissue banks specialize in recovering only a single kind of tissue; others handle combinations such as skin and bone or corneas and bone.

Competition Among Donor Organizations

An already confused situation is growing steadily more confused, because every organ donor is automatically a potential tissue donor. The federal government requires only that organ-procurement organizations cooperate with tissue banks. Some of these organizations are beginning to procure and distribute tissues in competition with existing tissue banks; others play favorites among competing tissue banks by notifying only one that a body will be available for tissue recovery once the organs have been removed. People involved in organ and tissue transplantation talk openly about "warfare."

One of the biggest battles is between the American Red Cross, which has started a national tissue service, and other procurement agencies and tissue banks. The Washington, D.C., chapter of the Red Cross recently tried to increase the fee that it charges for blood to any hospital that had not agreed to give tissue to the Red Cross, but then pulled back after the proposed contracts aroused concern in Congress. A 1984 federal statute prohibits the sale of human body parts but leaves tissue recovery and distribution largely unregulated. This absence of government regulation could easily lead to scandals down the road that would lessen the already pitiful donation rate; such scandals could focus, for example, on the absence of mandated safety standards or on possible abuse of the no-sale policy.

What happens to blood is instructive. In the United States today virtually all blood comes from altruistic donors. Yet, according to a series of articles in *The Philadelphia Inquirer*, blood banks, even nonprofit blood banks, buy and sell from one another more than a million pints of blood a year. The ultimate recipient of the blood could pay as much as $120 for a pint that was donated free of charge. This payment greatly exceeds the cost of processing and transporting the blood. From 1980 to 1988, according to the *Inquirer*, the Red Cross blood program alone generated profits of more than $300 million.

Great Demand, Meager Supply

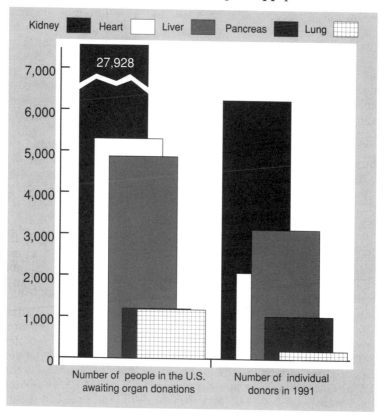

Source: United Network for Organ Sharing.

Current statutes do not regulate the potential for excessive earnings among organizations that procure, process, and distribute organs and tissues. A fully utilized body generates a substantial amount of medical business—the cost of transplanting the heart, kidneys, lungs, liver, and pancreas alone can reach $1 million—and the money cannot be ignored. The law prohibits donors or their heirs from receiving money for lifesaving body parts. But the surgeon, the hospital, even the chaplain who advises the grieving next of kin to make the donation, are all paid for their services. Although no one argues against fair payment, it's very likely that people will be less willing to donate parts of their bodies if they know that others will profit exorbitantly from the use of those parts. . . .

If cooperation and coordination are so obviously needed, why haven't they happened?

"In a system dependent on altruism," says Emanuel Thorne, an economist at Brooklyn College who is writing a book on the regulation of human organs and tissues, "organizations must be nonprofit. Were they profit-making, competition and takeovers might result in a rational system. However, because they're nonprofit, merges and acquisitions can't take place through market mechanisms, but must occur through politics and persuasion, which can take a long time. Moreover, the desired outcome is not at all assured."

Other difficult issues demand attention. Good medicine requires uniform data collection and the pooling of donor registries. Transplantation is a worldwide phenomenon. Organs and tissues increasingly cross national borders, although safety standards and reimbursement procedures vary from country to country. We need rules covering international trade and exchanges.

We also need to establish national safety and quality standards that guarantee the adequate testing of body parts for AIDS, hepatitis, and other infectious diseases. The Food and Drug Administration checks apples and aspirin but sets standards for only a few of the tissues and none of the organs that are transplanted directly from one body to another.

Low Supply Increases Costs

The cost of transplantation is another significant issue. According to UNOS, the average kidney transplant costs $25,000 to $30,000, a heart transplant $57,000 to $110,000, a liver transplant $135,000 to $230,000. (Pre- and post-transplant treatment, which can increase the cost significantly, have not been included in these estimates.) Permanent maintenance on immunosuppressive drugs may cost from $4,000 to $10,000 annually, and there will inevitably be fees for other medical care associated with the transplant. Transplantation, however, is often less costly than alternative treatments. For example, it costs more to keep a kidney patient on dialysis for a year than it does to buy a year's worth of post-transplant drugs. The Health Care Financing Administration estimates that a kidney transplant pays for itself in three or four years. Even allowing for such problems as the possible need for retransplantation, doubling the supply of kidneys could cut down on health-care costs by hundreds of millions of dollars.

Many transplant centers won't put a person on a waiting list for an organ unless that person can demonstrate the ability to pay for the transplant. Indeed, one of the most intractable problems for all of medicine pervades transplantation: the "green screen." Should anyone be denied a transplant for lack of the money? Many times access is denied for financial reasons, but not straightforwardly. For instance, in the case of bone-marrow transplantation, once the computer has identified potential matches, a patient may have to pay $175 to $600 to have each of them tested. Fees for the search and for subsequent laboratory work on donors also vary dramatically, and frequently exceed actual costs. Since insurance usually does not pay for testing anyone but the patient, families have had to mortgage homes or borrow from friends. When the money runs out, most marrow registries stop working. This situation persists even though, for some forms of leukemia, marrow transplantation may be less expensive than treatment with chemotherapy and/or radiation.

Roger Evans, of the Battelle-Seattle Research Center, calculates that 67 million people in the United States lack the insurance to cover the cost of a major organ transplant, such as that for a heart or lungs. They can donate organs and tissues but may be ineligible to receive them. This includes many residents of states such as Oregon and Wyoming, where Medicaid funding for major organ transplants is not available. "I do not believe you should ask anyone to participate as a donor when he can't participate as a recipient," says Terry Strom, an immunologist and professor of medicine at Harvard Medical School. "It becomes the rich buying health at the expense of the poor."

Government Must Intervene

Notwithstanding such hard issues, the ultimate reason reality lags so far behind medical possibility is the lack of federal effort. The government has for too long resisted establishing and funding a national policy to encourage an adequate supply—and the efficient and equitable use—of donated organs and tissues. And the public remains largely uninformed. Surgeons, still pioneering new types of transplantation, have pressed for action. Families unwilling to accept that no more can be done to save loved ones have formed marrow registries, mounted their own organ-procurement efforts, and tried to attract public attention. Most have come to the exasperated conclusion that something better must be possible. It is. In ways never before imagined, we can transform death and pain into life and hope.

"We are intentionally separating ourselves from what we believe has become an overly zealous medical and societal commitment to the endless perpetuation of life."

The Search for Organs Is Dehumanizing

Renée C. Fox and Judith P. Swazey

Renée C. Fox and Judith P. Swazey are social scientists long involved in the field of organ transplantation. In the following viewpoint, they say they are abandoning this area of work because "predatory obliviousness" is dehumanizing. They assert that in the quest to save and extend life, transplantation researchers and medical personnel have lost sight of what life actually means. Transplantation workers seek organs without questioning their source, and they seek to extend patients' lives without considering the effect of treatment on those lives, the authors contend.

As you read, consider the following questions:

1. What is meant by "the courage to fail" value system? Why do the authors deplore it?
2. What insight did their experiences in China give Fox and Swazey?
3. Why do the authors believe the current ardor for saving lives through organ replacement is excessive?

As journeyers into the field, participant observers, and chroniclers, we have been involved in the development of organ transplantation, the artificial kidney, and the artificial heart throughout most of their contemporaneous medical and social history and for many years of our working lives. Since 1951 (RCF) and 1968 (JPS) we have had the privileged opportunity to watch, from the inside, how dialysis and kidney, heart, and liver transplantation, which began as "desperate remedies for desperate patients," with certain "desperate[ly] hopeless" conditions [as described by Francis D. Moore], evolved into "nonexperimental," though far from ordinary, interventions to treat a wide gamut of end-stage diseases. During those years we have seen the range and combinations of different organs transplanted, the numbers performed, and the array of artificial organs designed increase dramatically, and we have charted at first hand the early phases of the drive to replace the human heart with a man-made device. . . .

Troubling Aspects of Organ Transplantation

Our decision to leave the field has been a complex one and a long time in the making. Over the past decade or so, we gradually recognized in ourselves the signs and symptoms of what we diagnosed as "participant-observer burnout"—akin to what we have witnessed over the years in some of the medical professionals immersed in the world of organ replacement efforts. Our burnout has its roots in the fact that there have been aspects of these efforts that we always have found especially troubling. Prominent among them have been some components of the "courage to fail" value system prevalent among transplantation and artificial organ pioneers. This ethos includes a classically American frontier outlook: heroic, pioneering, adventurous, optimistic, and determined. It also involves, however, a bellicose, "death is the enemy" perspective; a rescue-oriented and often zealous determination to maintain life at any cost; and a relentless, hubris-ridden refusal to accept limits. It is disturbing to witness, over and over, the travail and distress to which this outlook can subject patients. [As Leslie G. Reimer writes]:

I have often seen transplant surgeons, confronted with a clinical dilemma, begin to invoke a litany of names, like a litany of Roman Catholic saints [a transplant service chaplain reflects]: "It may be a real long shot," they say, "but remember Vernie and remember Toni and remember Carl and remember . . . and remember . . . and remember. . . ." (The litany, which always consists of patients who survived against seemingly impossible odds, is used as an argument for pressing on. There does not seem to be a parallel list that would argue for giving up.)

[Patricia M. Park writes]:

91

It is sometimes hard to meet the eyes of patients who have improved enough to have been moved to the regular postop floor and finally become alert enough to communicate their despair and disappointment. . . . Often, after entering the experience with such great hope, patients for whom transplantation has been a series of setbacks clearly articulate their feelings of betrayal: "No one ever told me it could be like this.". . .

Certainly they were told that there would be no guarantees, and that it would be hard, and that there would be setbacks—but probably not how hard, or what some of the worst-case scenarios could be. When they were told, "You have to have a transplant or you're going to die," they were left a very slim margin for decision making. These people need to know not only what it will be like not to be dying any more, but what it may be like to not live so well.

Another early source of unease was our conviction that if our society is to engage in such endeavors, we have a moral obligation to ensure equitable access to organ replacement. In the absence of such equity, we have observed again and again how specifically designated individuals have been privileged to obtain needed organs and funding for transplantation by wielding special emotional, media, political, and economic resources available to them, including, during the Reagan years, the power and resources of the presidency. [As Eike-Henner W. Kluge writes]:

Rather than focusing on conditions that ultimately are defensible in terms of equality and justice, . . . designated . . . person-specific . . . organ donation . . . ties access to an organ to the emotional appeal (or lack thereof) of the prospective recipient, the public relations skills of the physician[s] involved, of the next-of-kin, and of those who orchestrate the media campaign, and the financial abilities of everyone concerned to mount such a campaign in the first place. . . . [I]n effect [it] . . . singles out a specific individual and characterizes him or her as someone to whom an organ may be given independently of the established means of access. The assumption is that this person is ethically special; that he or she has some particular quality or characteristic that permits an exemption from the criteria that would otherwise apply to all.

Our decision to leave the field actually occurred in two phases. Our first attempt to do so turned out to be no more than a brief moratorium. From 1979-1982, partly under the aegis of the James Picker Foundation Program on the Human Qualities of Medicine, we conducted targeted field research for a book of essays that would be a sequel to *The Courage to Fail*. It was during the course of this work, as we immersed ourselves once more in the "lived-in reality" of the world of organ replacement endeavors, that we first seriously discussed leaving this field.

Many people and experiences from those years remain indelibly etched in our minds. It was the identified cases, relationships, and advances we were privileged to study first-hand that both powerfully bound us to the field for so long and, cumulatively, led us to withdraw from it. Among those still vivid images are the vista of an empty thoracic cavity awaiting the implantation of a heart and lungs from a brain-dead donor at Stanford; the sight of desperate parents and their tiny, dying children with huge eyes, bloated bellies, pale, lifeless hair, and ochre-colored skin, who had made pilgrimages to Dr. Thomas Starzl in Pittsburgh to plead for a liver transplant; and, in both of these settings, the first exuberant discussions about the miracles that were being wrought by the discovery of cyclosporine.

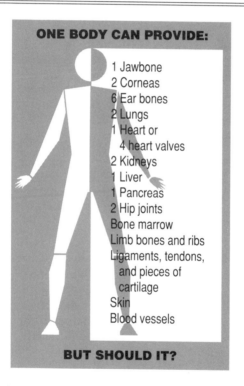

ONE BODY CAN PROVIDE:

1 Jawbone
2 Corneas
6 Ear bones
2 Lungs
1 Heart or
  4 heart valves
2 Kidneys
1 Liver
1 Pancreas
2 Hip joints
Bone marrow
Limb bones and ribs
Ligaments, tendons,
  and pieces of
  cartilage
Skin
Blood vessels

BUT SHOULD IT?

Source: *Time*, June 17, 1991.

Above all, it was the "identified lives"—the patients and families we came to know, some only slightly and others more intimately—that made us feel sadder and more anxious than we had in the past and filled us with painfully unanswerable questions of "why?". . . .

Six weeks of field research during the summer of 1981 in the People's Republic of China also had a powerful impact on us. During that era of the "four modernizations," China's medical workers had a collective commitment to "serving the patient" by progressively "scaling the heights" of modern medicine. It was part of a larger "golden dream" they shared with their compatriots about what science and technology might achieve for their country and its people. As part of this drive for medical modernization, hospitals in Tianjin were making their first forays into organ transplantation and chronic dialysis. As we watched these beginnings, we were vividly reminded of what Dr. Francis D. Moore termed the "black years" of renal transplantation in the United States—complete with the high mortality rate of patients and organs and what would now be considered in our country and in Western Europe excessive doses of corticosteroid immunosuppressive drugs, with all their side effects. Absorbed though we were by many features of our Chinese field experience, we were reluctant to "go through again" what RCF observed 40 years ago on the metabolic research ward of the Peter Bent Brigham Hospital in Boston, where renal transplantation and dialysis were pioneered. We also found ourselves in the peculiar cultural and ideological position of being more preoccupied than our hosts with the allocation of scarce resources dilemma that their dawning interest in transplantation, dialysis, intensive care medicine, and other advanced forms of Western medicine would pose for a country as poor as China, with a population of more than one billion persons and massive public health and primary care needs.

Bioethics Reflect American Values

China also provided us with a societal telescope through which, from a great historical, cultural, and physical distance, we were able to connect our thoughts about transplantation and dialysis with our growing sociological and moral concern about the state of American ideas, values, and beliefs, as epitomized by the predominant themes of bioethics a decade ago. In a comparative analysis of "medical morality" in China and bioethics in the United States, we wrote that

> if . . . bioethics is not just bioethics and is more than medical—if it is an indicator of the general state of American ideas, values and beliefs, of our collective self-knowledge, and our understanding of other societies' cultures—then there is every reason to be worried about who we are, what we have become, what we know, and where we are going in a greatly changed and changing society and world. . . .

In December 1982 . . . newspapers headlined the first implantation of a permanent total artificial heart by Dr. William DeVries and his colleagues at the University of Utah Medical Center. For the next 112 days, we and millions of others followed the drama of Dr. Barney Clark's life and death with a Jarvik-7 heart. However, because of the extensive case study we had made of the total artificial heart implant Dr. Denton Cooley attempted in 1969, the Barney Clark/William DeVries story had a magnetic effect on us, drawing us back into the field despite our resolve to leave it. And so, in June 1983 we found ourselves en route to Salt Lake City, for what we defined as a brief, one-time period of interviews and observations. However, more than five years passed before, in the fall of 1988, we completed what became a detailed and profoundly disquieting study of the development and use of the Jarvik heart. It was that research project and some of the participant observation experiences associated with it that brought our journeying into this field of medical research and therapeutic innovation to a definitive end.

Discomfort Concerning Promotion of Transplants

During the 1980s we also continued to monitor developments and issues in transplantation and dialysis, and our uneasiness about the attributes and side effects of organ replacement endeavors also continued to grow. . . . Through the ongoing process of self-scrutiny and self-analysis that participant observation also entails, we have recognized that our years in the field have made us more, rather than less emotionally and morally perturbable. For example, we found ourselves responding with stronger negative sentiments than in the past to such *déjà-vu* experiences as hearing some of the same transplanters who proclaimed the "cosmic" significance of cyclosporine now hail the newly discovered experimental immunosuppressive agent FK-506 as a once-in-a-lifetime miracle drug and learning that the Boy Scouts of America are offering a Donor Awareness Patch to induce scouts to talk to their families about organ donation. We reacted with concern to a proposal by Paul I. Terasaki, a pioneer of transplantation tissue-typing methods, that organ recipients "who are now enjoying a second chance at life, thanks to the compassionate generosity of the families of donors" be organized into "a trained . . . volunteer . . . self-perpetuating advocacy group" that could "take turns being on call to ask grieving families to consider organ donations, . . . visit hospital personnel . . . who . . . have limited personal contact with . . . a person who has been given life and health with someone else's heart, liver, or kidney," and "promote awareness" of the "mounting . . . need" for donations of cadaveric organs. When we read about multiple organ transplants, live-donor liver and lung transplants, conceiving

95

children to serve as bone marrow donors, the temporary use of diseased donor hearts, and about the merits of markets in human body parts—often referred to simply as "HBPs," we wondered, as did philosopher Daniel Callahan, "what kind of life" our values are driving us to seek, and if we can accept "limits to medical progress."

We are not therapeutic nihilists, nor do we lack appreciation for the impressive medical, surgical, and technological progress that has been made with transplants and artificial organs over the course of the past three decades, or just in the past 10 years. If anything, our in vivo historical relationship to their development has heightened our recognition of just how far they have advanced. Nor have we lost our capacity to respond with empathy to the "stories with happy endings," and to those that tragically never came to pass:

> For my family and me [a friend wrote us] the pain and grief of losing John was complicated by the bitter disappointment that we did not receive a heart in time to sustain his life. Intellectually, I know this is an incontrovertible fact. Emotionally, I know that we, his family, were his life and all of you are helping to sustain us. Perhaps, John *did* receive a heart. Although few of you knew him, you gave him yours.

But we have come to believe that the missionary-like ardor about organ replacement that now exists, the overidealization of the quality and duration of life that can ensue, and the seemingly limitless attempts to procure and implant organs that are currently taking place have gotten out of hand. In the words of a transplant nurse-specialist [Patricia M. Park], "perhaps the most important issue in a critical examination of transplantation involves the need and criteria for responsible decisions about when to stop, when to say 'enough is enough' to the transplant process."

An Unwillingness to Accept Death

In our view, the field of organ replacement now epitomizes a very different and powerful tendency in the American health care system and in the value and belief system of our society's culture: our pervasive reluctance to accept the biological and human condition limits imposed by the aging process to which we are all subject and our ultimate mortality. It seems to us that many of the current replacement endeavors represent an obdurate, publicly theatricalized refusal to accept these limitations. Physicians are morally guided by what the late Protestant theologian and ethicist Paul Ramsey called principles of "faithfulness" and "loyalty" not to abandon caring for their patients, particularly those who are dying. Ramsey also argued forcibly, however, that we "need . . . to discover the moral limits properly surrounding efforts to save life." With this conviction, we think that he would have joined us in questioning the enactment of the principle of faithfulness in the unremitting efforts of transplant surgeons to prevent the death of their patients by doing numerous retransplants if the donor organ "fails for any reason," because they believe [as Patricia Park notes] that "once a patient has had a transplant [they] have made a commitment that cannot be abandoned.". . .

One of the most urgent value questions that has emerged from our long professional immersion in the world of "spare parts" medicine is whether, as poverty, homelessness, and lack of access to health care increase in our affluent country, it is justifiable for American society to be devoting so much of its intellectual energy and human and financial resources to the replacement of human organs. We realize that in terms of the ways our society provides, allocates, and expends resources within the "medical commons," the aggregate volume and costs of organ replacements are a relatively small portion of medical care activities and expenditures. Nor, given the benefits that many patients may derive from transplants and artificial devices, do we suppose that all organ replacement endeavors should—or conceivably would—cease. We do believe, however, that all the professional and public consideration given to transplants and pursuits such as a permanent artificial heart and the societal value commitments that organ replacement epitomizes are helping to divert attention and human and financial resources away from far more basic and widespread public and individual health care needs in our society. . . .

In the final analysis, our departure from the field in the midst of such events is not only impelled by our need and desire to distance ourselves from them emotionally. It is also a value statement on our part. By our leave-taking we are intentionally separating ourselves from what we believe has become an overly zealous medical and societal commitment to the endless perpetuation of life and to repairing and rebuilding people through organ replacement—and from the human suffering and the social, cultural, and spiritual harm we believe such unexamined excess can, and already has, brought in its wake.

"It is only fair that patients who have not assumed equal responsibility for maintaining their health . . . should be treated differently."

Alcoholics Should Have Low Priority for Organ Transplants

Alvin H. Moss and Marvin Siegler

Many people believe that with the present shortage in organs for transplantation, a means must be found of allocating those available. One way, say some, is to rate potential recipients on the basis of their culpability for their own disease. A prime example is patients with alcoholism, which causes liver disease. In the following viewpoint, physicians Alvin H. Moss and Marvin Siegler, both affiliated with the Center for Clinical Medical Ethics at the University of Chicago, argue that no matter how one views alcoholism, to some degree the alcoholic is responsible for the liver disease that causes the need for a transplant. Consequently, other needy, less culpable patients should be considered for transplants before the alcoholic is.

As you read, consider the following questions:

1. What are the three main reasons, according to the authors, that alcoholics should be last on the list to receive needed liver transplants?
2. According to the authors, why is it just to single out alcoholics but not smokers, obese people, and others who have what might be called health-destructive traits?

From Alvin H. Moss and Marvin Siegler, "Should Alcoholics Compete Equally for Liver Transplantation?" *Journal of the American Medical Association* 261 (March 13, 1991): 1295-98. Copyright 1991, American Medical Association. Reprinted with permission.

Until recently, liver transplantation for patients with alcohol-related end-stage liver disease (ARESLD) was not considered a treatment option. Most physicians in the transplant community did not recommend it because of initial poor results in this population and because of a predicted high recidivism rate that would preclude long-term survival. In 1988, however, T.E. Starzl and colleagues reported 1-year survival rates for patients with ARESLD comparable to results in patients with other causes of end-stage liver disease (ESLD). Although the patients in the Pittsburgh series may represent a carefully selected population, the question is no longer Can we perform transplants in patients with alcoholic liver disease and obtain acceptable results? but Should we? This question is particularly timely since the Health Care Financing Administration (HCFA) has recommended that Medicare coverage for liver transplantation be offered to patients with alcoholic cirrhosis who are abstinent. The HCFA proposes that the same eligibility criteria be used for patients with ARESLD as are used for patients with other causes of ESLD, such as primary biliary cirrhosis and sclerosing cholangitis.

Should Patients with ARESLD Receive Transplants?

At first glance, this question seems simple to answer. Generally, in medicine, a therapy is used if it works and saves lives. But the circumstances of liver transplantation differ from those of most other lifesaving therapies, including long-term mechanical ventilation and dialysis, in three important respects:

Nonrenewable resource. First, although most lifesaving therapies are expensive, liver transplantation uses a nonrenewable, absolutely scarce resource—a donor liver. In contrast to patients with end-stage renal disease, who may receive either a transplant or dialysis therapy, every patient with ESLD who does not receive a liver transplant will die. This dire, absolute scarcity of donor livers would be greatly exacerbated by including patients with ARESLD as potential candidates for liver transplantation. In 1985, 63,737 deaths due to hepatic disease occurred in the United States, at least 36,000 of which were related to alcoholism, but fewer than 1,000 liver transplants were performed. Although patients with ARESLD represent more than 50% of the patients with ESLD, patients with ARESLD account for less than 10% of those receiving transplants. If patients with ARESLD were accepted for liver transplantation on an equal basis, as suggested by the HCFA, there would potentially be more than 30,000 additional candidates each year. (No data exist to indicate how many patients in the late stages of ARESLD would meet transplantation eligibility criteria.) In 1987, only 1,182 liver transplants were performed; in 1989, fewer than 2,000 were done. Even if all donor livers available were given to patients with ARESLD, it would not be feasible to provide transplants for even a small fraction of them. Thus, the dire, absolute nature of donor liver scarcity mandates that distribution be based on unusually rigorous standards—standards not required for the allocation of most other resources such as dialysis machines and ventilators, both of which are only *relatively* scarce.

Comparison with cardiac transplantation. Second, although a similar dire, absolute scarcity of donor hearts exists for cardiac transplantation, the allocational decisions for cardiac transplantation differ from those for liver transplantation. In liver transplantation, ARESLD causes more than 50% of the cases of ESLD; in cardiac transplantation, however, no one predominant disease or contributory factor is responsible. Even for patients with end-stage ischemic heart disease who smoked or who failed to adhere to dietary regimens, it is rarely clear that one particular behavior caused the disease. Also, unlike our proposed consideration for liver transplantation, a history of alcohol abuse is considered a contraindication and is a common reason for a patient with heart disease to be denied cardiac transplantation. Thus, the allocational decisions for heart transplantation differ from those for liver transplantation in two ways: determining a cause for end-stage heart disease is less certain, and patients with a history of alcoholism are usually rejected from heart transplant programs.

Expensive technology. Third, a unique aspect of liver transplantation is that it is an expensive technology that has become a target of cost containment in health care. It is, therefore, essential to maintain the approbation and support of the public so that organs continue to be donated under appropriate clinical circumstances—even in spite of the high cost of transplantation.

General Guideline Proposed

In view of the distinctive circumstances surrounding liver transplantation, we propose as a general guideline that patients with ARESLD should not compete equally with other candidates for liver transplantation. We are *not* suggesting that patients with ARESLD should *never* receive liver transplants. Rather, we propose that a priority ranking be established for the use of this dire, absolutely scarce societal resource and that patients with ARESLD be lower on the list than others with ESLD.

We realize that our proposal may meet with two immediate objections: (1) Some may argue that since alcoholism is a disease, patients with ARESLD should be considered equally for liver transplantation; (2) Some will question why patients with ARESLD should be singled out for discrimination, when the medical profession treats many patients who engage in behavior that causes their diseases. We will discuss these objections in turn.

We do not dispute the reclassification of alcoholism as a disease. Both hereditary and environmental factors contribute to alcoholism, and physiological, biochemical, and genetic markers have been associated with increased susceptibility. Identifying alcoholism as a disease enables physicians to approach it as they do other medical problems and to differentiate it from bad habits, crimes, or moral weaknesses. More important, identifying alcoholism as a disease also legitimizes medical interventions to treat it.

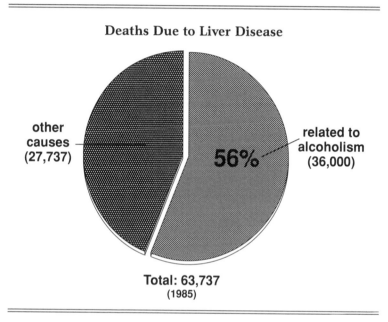

Deaths Due to Liver Disease

other causes (27,737)

56%

related to alcoholism (36,000)

Total: 63,737
(1985)

Alcoholism is a chronic disease, for which treatment is available and effective. More than 1.43 million patients were treated in 5,586 alcohol treatment units in the 12-month period ending October 30, 1987. One comprehensive review concluded that more than two-thirds of patients who accept therapy improve. Another cited four studies in which at least 54% of patients were abstinent a minimum of 1 year after treatment. A recent study of alcohol-impaired physicians reported a 100% abstinence rate an average of 33.4 months after therapy was initiated. In this study, physician-patients rated Alcoholics Anonymous, the largest organization of recovering alcoholics in the world, as the most important component of their therapy.

Like other chronic diseases—such as type I diabetes mellitus, which requires the patient to administer insulin over a lifetime—alcoholism requires the patient to assume responsibility for participating in continuous treatment. Two key elements are required to successfully treat alcoholism: the patient must accept his or her diagnosis and must assume responsibility for treatment. The high success rates of some alcoholism treatment programs indicate that many patients can accept responsibility for their treatment. ARESLD, one of the sequelae of alcoholism, results from 10 to 20 years of heavy alcohol consumption. The risk of ARESLD increases with the amount of alcohol consumed and with the duration of heavy consumption. In view of the quantity of alcohol consumed, the years, even decades, required to develop ARESLD, and the availability of effective alcohol treatment, attributing personal responsibility for ARESLD to the patient seems all the more justified. We believe, therefore, that even though alcoholism is a chronic disease, alcoholics should be held responsible for seeking and obtaining treatment that could prevent the development of late-stage complications such as ARESLD. Our view is consistent with that of Alcoholics Anonymous: alcoholics are responsible for undertaking a program for recovery that will keep their disease of alcoholism in remission.

Are We Discriminating Against Alcoholics?

Why should patients with ARESLD be singled out when a large number of patients have health problems that can be attributed to so-called voluntary health-risk behavior? Such patients include smokers with chronic lung disease; obese people who develop type II diabetes; some individuals who test positive for the human immunodeficiency virus; individuals with multiple behavioral risk factors (inattention to blood pressure, cholesterol, diet, and exercise) who develop coronary artery disease; and people such as skiers, motorcyclists, and football players who sustain activity-related injuries. We believe that the health care system should respond based on the actual medical needs of patients rather than on the factors (e.g., genetic, infectious, or behavioral) that cause the problem. We also believe that individuals should bear some responsibility—such as increased insurance premiums—for medical problems associated with voluntary choices. The critical distinguishing factor for treatment of ARESLD is the scarcity of the resource needed to treat it. The resources needed to treat most of these other conditions are only moderately or relatively scarce, and patients with these diseases or injuries can receive a share of the resources (i.e., money, personnel, and medication) roughly equivalent to their need. In contrast, there are insufficient donor livers to sustain the lives of all with ESLD who are in need. This difference permits us to make some discriminating choices—or to establish priorities—in selecting candidates for liver transplantation based on notions of fairness. In addition, this reasoning enables us to offer patients with alcohol-related medical and surgical problems their fair share of relatively scarce resources, such as blood products, surgical care, and intensive care beds, while still maintaining that their claim on donor livers is less compelling than the claims of others. . . .

Given a tragic shortage of donor livers, what is the fair or just way to allocate them? We suggest that patients who develop ESLD through no fault of their own (e.g., those with congenital biliary atresia or primary biliary cirrhosis) should have a higher priority in receiving a liver transplant than those whose liver disease results from failure to obtain treatment for alcoholism. In view of the dire, absolute scarcity of donor livers, we believe it is fair to hold people responsible for their choices, including decisions to refuse alcoholism treatment, and to allocate organs on this basis.

It is unfortunate but not unfair to make this distinction. When not enough donor livers are available for all who need one, choices have to be made, and they should be founded on one or more proposed principles of fairness for distributing scarce resources.

Should Any Alcoholics Be Considered for Transplantation?

Our proposal for giving lower priority for liver transplantation to patients with ARESLD does not completely rule out transplantation for this group. Patients with ARESLD who had not previously been offered therapy and who are now abstinent could be acceptable candidates. In addition, patients lower on the waiting list, such as patients with ARESLD who have been treated and are now abstinent, might be eligible for a donor liver in some regions because of the increased availability of donor organs there. Even if only because of these possible conditions for transplantation, further research is needed to determine which patients with ARESLD would have the best outcomes after liver transplantation.

Transplantation programs have been reluctant to provide transplants to alcoholics because of concern abut one unfavorable outcome: a high recidivism rate. Although the overall recidivism rate for the Pittsburgh patients was only 11.5%, in the patients who had been abstinent less than 6 months it was 43%. Also, compared with the entire group in which 1-year survival was 74%, the survival rate in this subgroup was lower, at 64%.

In the recently proposed Medicare criteria for coverage of liver transplantation, the HCFA acknowledged that the decision to insure patients with alcoholic cirrhosis "may be considered controversial by some." As if to counter possible objections, the

HCFA listed requirements for patients with alcoholic cirrhosis: patients must meet the transplant center's requirement for abstinence prior to liver transplantation and have documented evidence of sufficient social support to ensure both recovery from alcoholism and compliance with the regimen of immunosuppressive medication.

Further research should answer lingering questions about liver transplantation for ARESLD patients: Which characteristics of a patient with ARESLD can predict a successful outcome? How long is abstinence necessary to qualify for transplantation? What type of a social support system must a patient have to ensure good results? These questions are being addressed. Until the answers are known, we propose that further transplantation for patients with ARESLD be limited to abstinent patients who had not previously been offered alcoholism treatment and to abstinent treated patients in regions of increased donor liver availability and that it be carried out as part of prospective research protocols at a few centers skilled in transplantation and alcohol research.

Comment

Should patients with ARESLD compete equally for liver transplants? In a setting in which there is a dire, absolute scarcity of donor livers, we believe the answer is no. Considerations of fairness suggest that a first-come, first-served approach for liver transplantation is not the most just approach. Although this decision is difficult, it is only fair that patients who have not assumed equal responsibility for maintaining their health or for accepting treatment for a chronic disease should be treated differently. Considerations of public values and mores suggest that the public may not support liver transplantation if patients with ARESLD routinely receive more than half of the available donor livers. We conclude that since not all can live, priorities must be established and that patients with ARESLD should be given a lower priority for liver transplantation than others with ESLD.

"Patients who are sick because of alleged self-abuse ought not be grouped for discriminatory treatment."

Alcoholism Should Not Affect Organ Transplant Priorities

Carl Cohen, Martin Benjamin, and the Ethics and Social Impact Committee of the Transplant and Health Policy Center

Many people believe that because alcoholics could choose to end their addiction through willpower or treatment, they are not deserving of liver transplants that could save them from alcoholism-induced liver disease. In the following viewpoint, Carl Cohen and Martin Benjamin, both Ph.D.s and members of the Ethics and Social Impact Committee of the Transplant and Health Policy Center in Ann Harbor, Michigan, disagree with this belief. They and the other members of the committee argue that such a basis for allocating organs would be fallacious and discriminatory.

As you read, consider the following questions:

1. Why is the argument against giving alcoholics equal access to transplanted livers fallacious, according to the authors?
2. One basis often given for denying transplants to alcoholics is that the organs will be wasted on people who will simply go out and drink again. How do Cohen and Benjamin respond to this argument?
3. In order for a policy discriminating against alcoholics to be fair, what task do the authors say would have to be done?

From Carl Cohen, Martin Benjamin, and the Ethics and Social Impact Committee of the Transplant and Health Policy Center, Ann Arbor, Michigan, "Alcoholics and Liver Transplantation," *JAMA* 261 (March 13, 1991): 1299-1301. Copyright 1991, American Medical Association. Reprinted with permission.

Alcoholic cirrhosis of the liver—severe scarring due to the heavy use of alcohol—is by far the major cause of end-stage liver disease. For persons so afflicted, life may depend on receiving a new, transplanted liver. The number of alcoholics in the United States needing new livers is great, but the supply of available livers for transplantation is small. *Should those whose end-stage liver disease was caused by alcohol abuse be categorically excluded from candidacy for liver transplantation?* This question, partly medical and partly moral, must now be confronted forthrightly. Many lives are at stake.

Reasons of two kinds underlie a widespread unwillingness to transplant livers into alcoholics: First, there is a common conviction—explicit or tacit—that alcoholics are morally blameworthy, their condition the result of their own misconduct, and that such blameworthiness disqualifies alcoholics in unavoidable competition for organs with others equally sick but blameless. Second, there is a common belief that because of their habits, alcoholics will not exhibit satisfactory survival rates after transplantation, and that, therefore, good stewardship of a scarce lifesaving resource requires that alcoholics not be considered for liver transplantation. We examine both of these arguments.

The Moral Argument

A widespread condemnation of drunkenness and a revulsion for drunks lie at the heart of this public policy issue. Alcoholic cirrhosis—unlike other causes of end-stage liver disease—is brought on by a person's conduct, by heavy drinking. Yet if the dispute here were only about whether to treat someone who is seriously ill because of personal conduct, we would not say—as we do not in cases of other serious diseases resulting from personal conduct—that such conduct disqualifies a person from receiving desperately needed medical attention. Accident victims injured because they were not wearing seat belts are treated without hesitation; reformed smokers who become coronary bypass candidates partly because they disregarded their physicians' advice about tobacco, diet, and exercise are not turned away because of their bad habits. But new livers are a scarce resource, and transplanting a liver into an alcoholic may, therefore, result in death for a competing candidate whose liver disease was wholly beyond his or her control. Thus we seem driven, in this case unlike in others, to reflect on the weight given to the patient's personal conduct. And heavy drinking—unlike smoking, or overeating, or failing to wear a seat belt—is widely regarded as morally wrong.

Many contend that alcoholism is not a moral failing but a disease. Some authorities have recently reaffirmed this position, asserting that alcoholism is "best regarded as a chronic disease"

106

[as stated by F.L. Klerman in the *New England Journal of Medicine*]. But this claim cannot be firmly established and is far from universally believed. Whether alcoholism is indeed a disease, or a moral failing, or both, remains a disputed matter surrounded by intense controversy.

Even if it is true that alcoholics suffer from a somatic disorder, many people will argue that this disorder results in deadly liver disease only when coupled with a weakness of will—a weakness for which part of the blame must fall on the alcoholic. This consideration underlies the conviction that the alcoholic needing a transplanted liver, unlike a nonalcoholic competing for the same liver, is at least partly responsible for his or her need. Therefore, some conclude, the alcoholic's personal failing is rightly considered in deciding upon his or her entitlement to this very scarce resource.

Is this argument sound? We think it is not. Whether alcoholism is a moral failing, in whole or in part, remains uncertain. But even if we suppose that it is, it does not follow that we are justified in categorically denying liver transplants to those alcoholics suffering from end-stage cirrhosis. We could rightly preclude alcoholics from transplantation only if we assume that qualification for a new organ requires some level of moral virtue or is canceled by some level of moral vice. But there is absolutely no agreement—and there is likely to be none—about what constitutes moral virtue and vice and what rewards and penalties they deserve. The assumption that undergirds the moral argument for precluding alcoholics is thus unacceptable. Moreover, even if we could agree (which, in fact, we cannot) upon the kind of misconduct we would be looking for, the fair weighting of such a consideration would entail highly intrusive investigation into patients' moral habits—investigations universally thought repugnant. Moral evaluation is wisely and rightly excluded from all deliberations of who should be treated and how.

Others Are Not Judged

Indeed, we do exclude it. We do not seek to determine whether a particular transplant candidate is an abusive parent or a dutiful daughter, whether candidates cheat on their income taxes or their spouses, or whether potential recipients pay their parking tickets or routinely lie when they think it is in their best interests. We refrain from considering such judgments for several good reasons: (1) We have genuine and well-grounded doubts about comparative degrees of voluntariness and, therefore, *cannot pass judgment fairly.* (2) Even if we could assess degrees of voluntariness reliably, we *cannot know what penalties different degrees of misconduct deserve.* (3) *Judgments of this kind could not be made consistently in our medical system*—and a fundamental requirement of a fair system in allocating scarce resources is that it treat all in need of certain goods on the same standard, without unfair discrimination by group.

If alcoholics should be penalized because of their moral fault, then all others who are equally at fault in causing their own medical needs should be similarly penalized. To accomplish this, we would have to make vigorous and sustained efforts to find out whose conduct has been morally weak or sinful and to what degree. That inquiry, as a condition for medical care or for the receipt of goods in short supply, we certainly will not and should not undertake.

The unfairness of such moral judgments is compounded by other accidental factors that render moral assessment especially difficult in connection with alcoholism and liver disease. Some drinkers have a greater predisposition for alcohol abuse than others. And for some who drink to excess, the predisposition to cirrhosis is also greater; many grossly intemperate drinkers do not suffer grievously from liver disease. On the other hand, alcohol consumption that might be considered moderate for some may cause serious liver disease in others. It turns out, in fact, that the disastrous consequences of even low levels of alcohol consumption may be much more common in women than in men. Therefore, penalizing cirrhotics by denying them transplant candidacy would have the effect of holding some groups arbitrarily to a higher standard than others and would probably hold women to a higher standard of conduct than men.

Moral judgments that eliminate alcoholics from candidacy thus prove unfair and unacceptable. The alleged (but disputed) moral misconduct of alcoholics with end-stage liver disease does not justify categorically excluding them as candidates for liver transplantation.

Medical Argument

Reluctance to use available livers in treating alcoholics is due in some part to the conviction that, because alcoholics would do poorly after transplant as a result of their bad habits, good stewardship of organs in short supply requires that alcoholics be excluded from consideration.

This argument also fails, for two reasons: First, it fails because the premise—that the outcome for alcoholics will invariably be poor relative to other groups—is at least doubtful and probably false. Second, it fails because, even if the premise were true, it could serve as a good reason to exclude alcoholics only if it were an equally good reason to exclude other groups having a prognosis equally bad or worse. But equally low survival rates have not excluded other groups; fairness therefore requires that this group not be categorically excluded either.

In fact, the data regarding the posttransplant histories of alcoholics are not yet reliable. Evidence gathered in 1984 indicated that the 1-year survival rate for patients with alcoholic cirrhosis was well below the survival rate for other recipients of liver transplants, excluding those with cancer. But a 1988 report, with a larger (but still small) sample number, shows remarkably good results in alcoholics receiving transplants: 1-year survival is 73.2%—and of 35 carefully selected (and possibly nonrepresentative) alcoholics who received transplants and lived 6 months or longer, only two relapsed into alcohol abuse. Liver transplantation, it would appear, can be a very sobering experience. Whether this group continues to do as well as a comparable group of nonalcoholic liver recipients remains uncertain. But the data, although not supporting the broad inclusion of alcoholics, do suggest that medical considerations do not now justify categorically excluding alcoholics from liver transplantation.

No Reason to Exclude Alcoholics

Experts are coming to recognize that there is no moral or medical reason to exclude alcoholics for liver transplantation just because they are alcoholics. The limiting factors seem to be whether candidates are mentally or physically impaired from other well known complications of alcoholism that damage the brain, heart and blood system.

Several leaders have hammered away at the inconsistencies and the unique requirement from alcoholics that they abstain from alcohol. Those seeking transplants for other diseases are not held to the same standards. Smokers who need heart transplants are told to quit smoking, but they are not generally deprived of a suitable organ if they are unable to comply. . . .

Many would side with Dr. George D. Lundberg, the editor of the *Journal of the American Medical Association*, who said that if he had several possible recipients for a single organ, he would try to decide who was the most deserving recipient. He said he held to the view he expressed in an editorial in 1983: "If I had one liver to transplant and 50,000 possible recipients, I wouldn't let the fact that a great creative genius might drink deter me from giving him or her a needed new liver to allow another 30 years of creativity."

Lawrence K. Altman, *The New York Times*, April 3, 1990.

A history of alcoholism is of great concern when considering liver transplantation, not only because of the impact of alcohol abuse upon the entire system of the recipient, but also because the life of an alcoholic tends to be beset by general disorder. Returning to heavy drinking could ruin a new liver, although probably not for years. But relapse into heavy drinking would quite likely entail the inability to maintain the routine of multiple medication, daily or twice-daily, essential for immunosuppression and survival. As a class, alcoholic cirrhotics may therefore prove to have substantially lower survival rates after receiving transplants. All such matters should be weighed, of course. But none of them gives any solid reason to exclude alcoholics from consideration categorically.

Moreover, even if survival rates for alcoholics selected were much lower than normal—a supposition now in substantial doubt—what could fairly be concluded from such data? Do we exclude from transplant candidacy members of other groups known to have low survival rates? In fact we do not. Other things being equal, we may prefer not to transplant organs in short supply into patients afflicted, say, with liver cell cancer, knowing that such cancer recurs not long after a new liver is implanted. Yet in some individual cases we do it. Similarly, some transplant recipients have other malignant neoplasms or other conditions that suggest low survival probability. Such matters are weighed in selecting recipients, but they are insufficient grounds to categorically exclude an entire group. This shows that the argument for excluding alcoholics based on survival probability rates alone is simply not just.

The Arguments Distinguished

In fact, the exclusion of alcoholics from transplant candidacy probably result from an intermingling, perhaps at times confusion, of the moral and medical arguments. But if the moral argument indeed does not apply, no combination of it with probable survival rates can make it applicable. Survival data, carefully collected and analyzed, deserve to be weighed in selecting candidates. These data do not come close to precluding alcoholics from consideration. Judgments of blameworthiness, which ought to be excluded generally, certainly should be excluded when weighing the impact of those survival rates. Some people with a strong antipathy to alcohol abuse and abusers may without realizing it, be relying on assumed unfavorable data to support fixed moral judgment. The argument must be untangled. Actual results with transplanted alcoholics must be considered without regard to moral antipathies.

The upshot is inescapable: there are no good grounds at present—moral or medical—to disqualify a patient with end-stage liver disease from consideration for liver transplantation simply because of a history of heavy drinking. . . .

Patients who are sick because of alleged self-abuse ought not be grouped for discriminatory treatment—unless we are prepared to develop a detailed calculus of just deserts for health care based on good conduct. Lack of sympathy for those who bring serious disease upon themselves is understandable, but the temptation to institutionalize that emotional response must be tempered by our inability to apply such considerations justly and by our duty *not* to apply them unjustly. In the end, some patients with alcoholic cirrhosis may be judged, after careful evaluation, as good risks for a liver transplant.

Objection and Reply

Providing alcoholics with transplants may present a special "political" problem for transplant centers. The public perception of alcoholics is generally negative. The already low rate of organ donation, it may be argued, will fall even lower when it becomes known that donated organs are going to alcoholics. Financial support from legislatures may also suffer. One can imagine the effect on transplantation if the public were to learn that the liver of a teenager killed by a drunken driver had been transplanted into an alcoholic patient. If selecting even a few alcoholics as transplant candidates reduces the number of lives saved overall, might that not be good reason to preclude alcoholics categorically?

No. The fear is understandable, but excluding alcoholics cannot be rationally defended on that basis. Irresponsible conduct attributable to alcohol abuse should not be defended. No excuses should be made for the deplorable consequences of drunken behavior, from highway slaughter to familial neglect and abuse. But alcoholism must be distinguished from those consequences; not all alcoholics are morally irresponsible, vicious, or neglectful drunks. If there is a general failure to make this distinction, we must strive to overcome that failure, not pander to it.

Public confidence in medical practice in general, and in organ transplantation in particular, depends on the scientific validity and moral integrity of the policies adopted. Sound policies will prove publicly defensible. Shaping present health care policy on the basis of distorted public perceptions or prejudices will, in the long run, do more harm than good to the process and to the reputation of all concerned.

Approximately one in every 10 Americans is a heavy drinker, and approximately one family in every three has at least one member at risk for alcoholic cirrhosis. The care of alcoholics and the just treatment of them when their lives are at stake are matters a democratic polity may therefore be expected to act on with concern and reasonable judgment over the long run. The allocation of organs in short supply does present vexing moral problems; if thoughtless or shallow moralizing would cause some to respond very negatively to transplanting livers into alcoholic cirrhotics, that cannot serve as good reason to make such moralizing the measure of public policy.

We have argued that there is now no good reason, either moral or medical, to preclude alcoholics categorically from consideration for liver transplantation. We further conclude that it would therefore be unjust to implement that categorical preclusion simply because others might respond negatively if we do not.

Periodical Bibliography

The following articles have been selected to supplement the diverse views presented in this chapter.

American Health Consultants	"Organ Donation Proposed from Legally Alive Infants," *Medical Ethics Advisor*, May 1992.
American Health Consultants	"Proposals to Increase Supply of Organs Cause Concern," *Medical Ethics Advisor*, August 1991.
Bob Brecher	"The Kidney Trade: Or, the Customer Is Always Wrong," *Journal of Medical Ethics*, September 1990.
Courtney S. Campbell	"Body, Self, and the Property Paradigm," *Hastings Center Report*, September/October 1992.
Christine Gorman	"Matchmaker, Find Me a Match," *Time*, June 17, 1991.
J. Harvey	"Paying Organ Donors," *Journal of Medical Ethics*, September 1990.
Peter MacPherson	"Organ Transplants: Improving the Harvest," *Governing*, January 1993.
Madeline Marget	"The Need to Preserve Hope," *Commonweal*, March 27, 1992.
SSM Health Care System	"Is It Ethical to Compel People to 'Do Good'?" *Issues*, September/October 1990. Available from SSM Health Care System, 1031 Bellevue Ave., St. Louis, MO 63117.
Thomas Starzl	"Interview," *Omni*, September 1990.
Bernard Teo	"Organs for Transplantation: The Singapore Experience," *Hastings Center Report*, November/December 1991.
Emanuel D. Thorne	"Tissue Transplants: The Dilemma of the Body's Growing Value," *The Public Interest*, Winter 1990.

What Ethics Should Guide Fetal Tissue Research?

Biomedical Ethics

Chapter Preface

In the mid-1980s researchers believed they were on the path to alleviating, possibly even curing, debilitating diseases such as Parkinson's and Alzheimer's. Their research involved the implantation of fetal tissues into certain organs of the patient. Why fetal tissues? Researchers found that the body is more likely to accept fetal tissue than similar tissue from a fully developed person.

Because much of the fetal tissue used in such research comes from aborted fetuses, its use is controversial. Many researchers believe the promise offered by fetal tissue transplantation outweighs the procedure's ethical or moral considerations. If the research is successful, they argue, millions of people will be saved the devastating effects of degenerative diseases. Other researchers and ethicists, however, assert that the procedure is far from moral. Using the tissues and organs of aborted fetuses, they say, encourages the questionable practice of abortion.

In 1988, because of strong lobbying by opponents of fetal tissue research, the National Institutes of Health forbade further funding of such research with federal money. In effect, nearly all research in this area was halted. Although many people continued to lobby against this ban, it held until early 1993 when newly inaugurated president Bill Clinton decreed that such research could begin again.

Despite the renewal of fetal tissue research, experimentation, and transplantation, controversy continues to rage over this issue. The authors in the following chapter debate some of the questions relating to fetal tissue research.

"None of the alternatives [to fetal tissue obtained in induced abortions] offer a reasonable source of fetal tissue for transplantation research."

Fetal Tissue Is Essential to Medical Research

Daniel J. Garry, Arthur L. Caplan, Dorothy E. Vawter, and Warren Kearney

The four authors of the following viewpoint, Daniel J. Garry, Arthur L. Caplan, Dorothy E. Vawter, and Warren Kearney, are bioethicists and/or physicians. Garry and Kearney practice medicine out of Minneapolis hospitals. Caplan is the director of the University of Minnesota's Center for Biomedical Ethics, and Vawter is a research associate there. The four argue that fetal tissue is essential to researchers seeking ways to ameliorate or cure several debilitating diseases. The authors assert that despite the ethical misgivings of some critics, tissue from induced abortions must be made available to researchers because other potential sources (miscarriages and ectopic pregnancies, for example) are not viable alternatives.

As you read, consider the following questions:

1. What qualities make fetal tissue ideal for some transplants, according to the authors?
2. What common reasons make tissues from ectopic pregnancies and spontaneous abortions unsuitable for transplantation, according to the authors?
3. Do the authors have any misgivings about using human fetal tissues? Explain.

Daniel J. Garry, Arthur L. Caplan, Dorothy E. Vawter, and Warren Kearney, "Are There Really Alternatives to the Use of Fetal Tissue from Elective Abortions in Transplantation Research?" *The New England Journal of Medicine* 327 (November 26, 1992): 1592-95. Reprinted with permission.

Human fetal tissue has been described as having tremendous plasticity and availability, and as possibly being less prone to rejection than adult tissue. These properties have led many researchers to consider it a possible source of transplantable tissue for patients with incurable debilitating diseases, such as diabetes mellitus and Parkinson's, Alzheimer's, and Huntington's diseases.

The use of human fetal tissue in research involving transplantation in human recipients has become the center of a heated controversy in the United States. . . .

What is remarkable and disturbing about the current debate is that it remains almost completely devoid of information about alternative sources of fetal tissue. If there are scientific reasons that seriously limit the chances that tissue derived from ectopic pregnancies, spontaneously aborted fetuses, stillborn fetuses, or extraembryonic tissue could serve as an alternative to tissue obtained from electively aborted fetuses, then there is very little reason, other than politics, to fund only research using tissue from these sources. Oddly, this is precisely the situation that now exists. None of the alternatives offer a reasonable source of fetal tissue for transplantation research.

Ectopic Pregnancies

A number of writers have suggested that ectopic pregnancy is a practical and ethically uncontroversial source of human fetal tissue. In an ectopic pregnancy, the conceptus is implanted outside the uterus, with the most common sites being the oviduct (in more than 95 percent of cases), the abdominal cavity, and the ovary. Such a situation does not result in a successful pregnancy or delivery.

Ectopic pregnancies occur at a rate of 16.8 per 1000 reported pregnancies. In 1987 there were 88,000 ectopic pregnancies in the United States. Some tubal pregnancies resolve naturally or abort spontaneously. It has been estimated that approximately 60 percent of ectopic pregnancies abort spontaneously early in the first trimester. In one study, women with diagnosed ectopic pregnancy were hospitalized for one week to monitor their clinical symptoms and were then discharged and followed as outpatients, with daily clinical examinations and determinations of serum human chorionic gonadotropin levels. The ectopic pregnancy resolved spontaneously in 64 percent; the remaining patients required surgical intervention. Spontaneously aborted ectopic pregnancies rarely produce fetal tissue that is recognizable or viable in culture. Even when they do, the tissue has almost always been ischemic for days before its expulsion.

Ectopic pregnancies that do not abort spontaneously become clinically apparent before the ninth week of gestation. Surgical removal of the ectopic products of conception frequently reveals the absence of any fetal tissue. In one study of 65 ectopic pregnancies, 33 specimens (51 percent) were morphologically abnormal: 18 of these specimens had an intact chorionic sac with no recognizable embryo, 8 had no recognizable organ differentiation, and 7 had systemic abnormalities (i.e., spina bifida, microcephaly, or severe growth retardation). These findings are consistent with a previous report of 44 specimens from ectopic pregnancies, 28 of which (64 percent) were morphologically abnormal. Yet another recent study of 53 proved ectopic pregnancies revealed 42 specimens (79 percent) to be lacking in fetal tissue or grossly abnormal. In this study, only two of the ectopic pregnancies were viable (i.e., had evidence of myocardial contractility), as observed with ultrasound before the surgical removal of the ectopic conceptus.

Ectopic pregnancy is also linked with a high incidence of hemorrhage, which is associated with probable episodic anoxia to the ectopic fetus. Morphologic examination of 242 ectopic pregnancies revealed that the dilation of the oviduct was due primarily to intratubal hemorrhage. In most cases the growing ectopic fetus had penetrated the wall of the oviduct and assumed an extratubal location. P.F. Brenner et al. describe tubal rupture in 297 of 300 ectopic pregnancies, or 99 percent of women who were examined by laparotomy. Tubal rupture casts doubt on the viability and normality of tissues taken from fetuses that develop under such circumstances.

The only circumstance in which tissue from an ectopic pregnancy may be viable occurs when fetal myocardial contractility is observed before surgical removal. Such cases are exceedingly rare and are likely to become more so in the future. Nonsurgical therapy is currently being studied as treatment for ectopic pregnancy in order to preserve fertility. Methotrexate and mifepristone (RU 486), an antiprogestogen, have been administered with some degree of success. Pharmacologic advances are likely to reduce or eliminate the already tiny number of ectopic pregnancies that might yield normal, viable fetal tissue.

Spontaneous Abortion

Spontaneously aborted fetuses are another source of tissue often suggested by those who advocate federal funding for tissue banks that do not use fetal tissue from elective abortions. Some authors and government officials claim that such fetuses are both plentiful and ethically appropriate for use in transplantation.

A spontaneous abortion is the unintentional delivery of an embryo or fetus that has died in utero before the 20th week of gestation. The causes include major chromosomal or other lethal defects in the fetus, infections (e.g., syphilis, rubella, or mycoplasma), and maternal diseases (e.g., diabetes millitus). Tissue obtained from a fetus that has spontaneously aborted for any of these reasons would hardly be acceptable for transplantation.

Fetal Tissue Needed

Medical research using human fetal tissue offers considerable promise. Fetal liver, thymus, pancreatic and neural tissues have been transplanted in an attempt to combat Parkinson's, diabetes and twenty or so other diseases. . . . Human fetal tissue is especially suited for such transplants because it grows rapidly and adapts readily (as it would have done in the womb). Also, the fetal immune system is relatively undeveloped, so fetal tissue is less likely than mature tissue to trigger an immunological response in the recipient that leads to rejection. Transplantation is not the only promising avenue of research. Cell lines derived from fetal tissue are valuable in the laboratory for studying species-specific viruses such as cytomegalovirus and human immunodeficiency virus-type 1 (HIV-1).

Glenn C. Graber, *Priorities*, Summer 1992.

Rare causes of spontaneous abortion, such as uterine anomalies (e.g., an incompetent cervix), multiple pregnancy, and intrauterine fetal death as a result of motor vehicle accidents or other trauma (most frequently resulting in fracture of the fetal skull), may produce "normal" fetal tissue. But such tissue is not necessarily viable.

There are few data on the number of spontaneous abortions each year in the United States. Of all recognizable pregnancies, an estimated 15 to 20 percent, or 750,000, end in spontaneous abortion in the first trimester. Chromosomal abnormality is the most frequent cause of such abortions, accounting for 60 percent. In general, the earlier the gestational age at the time of spontaneous abortion, the more likely that its cause is a chromosomal abnormality. Trisomies account for 60 percent of all such abnormalities in fetuses aborted spontaneously during the first trimester. Turner's syndrome (in which the fetus has a 45,X karyotype) and polyploidy account for 20 percent each.

Investigators studying the association between certain diseases and chromosomal abnormalities may find spontaneously aborted fetuses the best source of tissue for their purposes. But chromosomally abnormal tissue is not optimal or even acceptable for transplantation, since its growth, development, and function are unreliable.

Most spontaneous abortions occur in the first trimester and

are preceded by fetal death in utero. Initially, there is hemorrhage, followed by tissue necrosis and inflammation at or near the site of implantation. The conceptus may then become detached from the uterine wall, and with subsequent uterine contractions the products of conception may be expelled, typically two or three weeks later. Any products that are not expelled must be surgically removed. This long delay in the expulsion of the dead fetus from the body renders the tissue of nearly all spontaneously aborted fetuses unsuitable for transplantation.

Furthermore, most such fetuses are incomplete specimens with no recognizable fetal tissue. One large study recently monitored 1025 spontaneous abortions over a 12-month period and found that 77 percent did not contain recognizable fetal tissue. Although 23 percent of the spontaneously aborted pregnancies yielded identifiable fetal tissue, only 3.8 percent produced a recognizable fetus that was not fragmented, stunted, or with some other obvious anomaly.

Miscarriages Produce Unusable Tissue

If 3.8 percent of the approximately 750,000 pregnant women known to abort spontaneously each year in the United States produce a normal fetus, then the tissue from approximately 28,500 spontaneously aborted fetuses could theoretically be used for transplantation if the fetuses were expelled or surgically removed within hours of fetal death. But even this number is not an accurate indication of the number of fetuses available as a result of spontaneous abortion. Most spontaneously aborted fetuses die in utero two to three weeks before expulsion. In addition, most spontaneous abortions occur outside a health care setting. As a result, the fetal tissue is often contaminated with environmental bacteria and is separated from the appropriate culture medium for many hours. Even in the rare cases in which a spontaneously aborted fetus yields viable fetal tissue, the high rate of major chromosomal anomalies associated with such abortions makes it obligatory to test such tissue for chromosomal abnormalities. Chromosomal analysis requires approximately 10 days and would probably necessitate the preservation of the fetal tissue until the test results became available. Thus, the quality of the tissue might be further compromised by the need for lengthy storage while its condition is established. Finally, it is not known how many women would consent to the use of tissue from their spontaneous abortions. But the unexpected and often tragic circumstances surrounding the event make it likely that some would refuse.

In sum, obtaining tissue from a dead fetus after a spontaneous abortion is morally acceptable to most people because the fetal death is perceived as tragic, not immoral. However, the overwhelming number of spontaneous abortions occur outside a medical setting, involve a fetus with chromosomal or other abnormalities, yield an incompletely developed fetus, or yield only nonviable tissue (because of the two-to-three-week period of ischemia before expulsion). And some women will not allow fetal remains to be used for transplantation research. Thus, spontaneously aborted fetuses are not reliable or safe as a source of normal, viable fetal tissue.

Stillbirths

Stillbirth is defined by the National Center for Health Statistics as fetal death in or after the 20th week of gestation. In 1983 there were approximately 30,280 stillbirths in the United States. In a typical clinical scenario, a woman who has had an uneventful pregnancy might present to the outpatient clinic anxiously reporting that she has been unaware of fetal movement for one or two days. Sonographic examination would reveal fetal death. After the delivery of the stillbirth, postmortem examination often reveals a macerated fetus.

An analysis of 765 consecutive stillbirths showed the identifiable causes of fetal death to be anoxia (in 43 percent), hemorrhage (16 percent), congenital anomalies (10 percent), diabetes mellitus (5 percent), and trauma (2 percent). Other studies report that in approximately half the cases the cause of death is unknown.

After a fetus dies in utero, it is usually retained for a time and then delivered spontaneously. A recent review of the literature indicates that at least 75 percent of women go into labor spontaneously within two weeks of fetal death and that the rest deliver within another two weeks. Tissue from these fetuses is not viable. Attempts to culture tissue from stillborn fetuses have rarely succeeded.

Moreover, stillbirths do not yield tissue that is at the stage of development required for most transplants. Neural tissue, for example, must usually be obtained from fetuses of less than 12 weeks' gestational age. The procurement of tissue from stillbirths raises little ethical concern. In fact, in some states the Uniform Anatomical Gift Act explicitly permits the use of tissue from stillbirths in transplantation. In practice, however, getting informed consent from a woman just after a stillbirth is problematic. In sum, the source that raises the least ethical concern is unlikely to provide any tissue suitable for transplantation research.

Extraembryonic Tissue

Extraembryonic tissue—that is, the placenta and yolk sac—can provide some fetal tissue for transplantation. Such tissue can be obtained from living fetuses early in gestation by diagnostic procedures such as chorionic-villus sampling and amniocentesis. Alternatively, extraembryonic tissue may be available after an abortion.

Fetal tissue from a placenta has unique characterics. Placental trophoblasts lack major histocompatibility complex Class II antigens and may therefore be less immunogenic than embryonic tissue. Although placental tissue cannot provide fetal islet or neuronal cells, it can be used to develop certain cell lines that might conceivably be engineered genetically to produce insulin or neurotransmitters such as dopamine.

Yolk-sac tissue is a well-recognized source of hematopoietic stem cells. This tissue could be proliferated in vitro, cryopreserved, and later transplanted into recipients with hematologic disorders. Conceivably, yolk-sac tissue may be an alternative to the use of fetal-liver cells in transplantation.

Extraembryonic tissue can be used for transplantation in only a limited number of patients, such as those with hematologic defects. The use of extraembryonic tissue obtained by diagnostic testing of living fetuses raises ethical questions. It is unknown what volume of tissue is safe to remove during such procedures. Nor is there agreement about how consent for the use of this tissue should be obtained. Many would deem it unethical to undertake procedures with the sole intention of removing extraembryonic tissue for research or transplantation.

Alternative Sources or Political Diversion?

Ectopic pregnancies, spontaneously aborted fetuses, and still-births would at best be rare and unpredictable sources of normal, viable fetal tissue. Since the availability of useful tissue from any of these sources is unpredictable, it is difficult for researchers and transplantation surgeons to make optimal use of it when it becomes available. Moreover, the incidence of abnormality associated with these categories of tissue is extraordinarily high. As a result, the transplantation of tissue obtained from these sources may expose the recipients to higher risks than those associated with other possible sources of fetal tissue, and the use of such tissue may slow or interfere with scientific progress in understanding the efficacy of fetal-tissue transplants. The only advantage to using these types of tissue is that some perceive them as raising less ethical concern with respect to tissue procurement. Even if this were true, the moral advantages perceived by some would not seem to outweigh the disadvantages to scientific progress and the increased risks imposed on human subjects that are entailed in the use of these types of fetal tissue.

"The public perception that fetal cell transplantation is a proven, if experimental, technology isn't true."

Fetal Tissue's Efficacy Has Not Been Proven

Michael Fumento

Journalist Michael Fumento reports on science and economic issues for *Investor's Business Daily* in Los Angeles. He has also written articles on health issues for various publications and is the author of the book *The Myth of Heterosexual AIDS*. In the following viewpoint, Fumento argues that the results of fetal tissue research are far from persuasive. He cites evidence showing that such research has had mixed or poor results, and he points to new therapies that promise to surpass fetal cell transplantation in their efficacy. Considering both scientific and moral concerns, he says, researchers would do well to abandon fetal tissue research.

As you read, consider the following questions:

1. Fumento suggests that certain scientific and popular publications have been "boosterish" advocates in their reports on fetal tissue research. What evidence does he use to support this assertion?
2. The author cites the work of Dr. William Landau. What explanation does Landau give for the seeming success of fetal tissue implants on Parkinson patients?
3. What are some of the negative side effects the author suggests could result from fetal tissue implantation?

Not long ago, brain transplants seemed the stuff of cheap science fiction. The scientific consensus has long been that once a brain begins to go, there is no restoring it, that the billions of cells the brain has at birth gradually die off through life and are not replaced, regardless of whether one killed the cells through drinking, boxing, or simply growing older. But it now appears possible that, for victims of Parkinson's, Alzheimer's, and other brain diseases, fresh cells grafted into the brain can stimulate functions once thought lost. Cells taken from fetuses are preferred for such grafts for two major reasons: they proliferate, and they are less likely to be rejected by the cell recipient.

Fetal transplants could herald a new age in medicine, with benefits to victims of Huntington's disease, amyotrophic lateral sclerosis (Lou Gehrig's disease), Alzheimer's disease, strokes, blindness, and traumatic brain injury. They could also usher in a Brave New World. According to ethicist Arthur Caplan of the Hastings Center outside New York: "The use of fetuses as organ and tissue donors is a ticking time bomb of bioethics.". . .

Abortion and Fetal Ethics

"Unconscionable" is a term used by both sides in the fetal tissue debate. There seems to be no argument over the use of tissue obtained after a miscarriage; in such cases, the woman's proxy consent is comparable to the consent of a parent to organ or tissue donation from her child. But the wide-scale use of miscarriages is impractical. Collection of fetuses is difficult, and whatever killed the fetus can cause any number of problems with the brain tissue. The real debate is over elective abortions. . . .

Then there are those like Dr. William Landau, head of the Department of Neurology at Washington University in St. Louis, who thinks that the talk about ethics is all quite superfluous for one reason: the public perception that fetal cell transplantation is a proven, if experimental, technology isn't true. "This is absolute science fiction," says Landau. "There's no evidence that the brain can be transplanted functionally in an animal and it will work. The brain is a unique organ that doesn't regenerate new cells and this isn't going to be changed by anybody."

Some of what lies behind this perception appears to be advocacy. Even science journals have given in to boosterism. *Science* stated in a 1990 news article: "The results of such surgery are undeniably dramatic: Patients whose movements have been impaired for decades by the disorder have been returned to near normal functioning by dopamine-secreting tissues transplanted directly into their brains. And yet, the method has been politically and ethically sensitive."

Contrast that with the subtitle of an editorial in the August

1990 *British Medical Journal*: "More Patients Have Probably Been Harmed Than Helped, So Far," or the 1988 *Science News* article, "Fetal Cell Transplants Show Few Benefits." Says Dartmouth Associate Professor of Neurology Richard Harbaugh, "I think if you went back through thirty years of *Science* and tried to find another single patient case report, unblinded and uncontrolled, you couldn't do it. For something like this to be in *Science* is unheard of."

The hype may also have a political bent. In order to circumvent the FDA [Food and Drug Administration's] ban on the French abortifacient RU-486, abortion activists have readily grabbed at whispers of evidence that the drug "may" have properties that "may" make it effective against AIDS, cancer, and other diseases. Those arguing for less destruction of the Brazilian rain forests are now advertising that among the unknown plants therein "may" be a cure for AIDS and cancer. In the broadest sense of the word "may," these assertions "may" prove correct. But they do not reflect scientific trial and error so much as the reality that for every disease you claim you "may" have a cure for, you pull in a constituency.

Temptation to Exaggerate

Landau has no doubt that the temptation to exaggerate has been succumbed to. He says he has no ethical problems with using aborted fetuses for either experimentation or therapy—the real ethical problem is chopping holes in the brains of people who are not terminally ill when adequate animal studies have not even been performed. Writing in the May 1990 issue of *Neurology*, Landau said, "This is not just an issue of bent statistics. Rather, it is one of lost scientific principles."

Landau, who has researched Parkinsonism for thirty years, is well aware of the pressures on researchers to produce positive results. He accuses no fetal cell researchers of trying to deceive anyone—other than perhaps themselves. He says that researchers are not following basic scientific procedures, and believes that Parkinson's patients benefit simply from surgical damage in the brain that is made in the course of transplants:

> There's no evidence that the transplant experiments in animals or man show anything other than the benefits of these cuts. . . . It's my belief, based on my knowledge of biology, that it won't work. The likelihood that tissue will make a functional connection with the way other cells work is improbable. The circuitry of the brain is complex. It's not like putting a piece of liver into another liver. There are different types of tissue in the brain. I can't conceive of how infantile brain cells stuck in an adult brain will make proper connections.

On May 10, [1992] the *Los Angeles Times* ran an editorial entitled "More Proof, Though None Is Needed," urging President

Bush to lift the fetal transplant ban. It based its argument on two studies released a few days earlier at a San Diego convention updating the fetal cell transplant experiments in Colorado and at Yale. The editorial reported that some of the patients given cells had improved, without noting that the control patients in the Yale study—those who had not received fetal cells —had also improved, a result that calls into question the effectiveness of fetal cell transplants. It also neglected to mention a study headed up by New York University neurosurgeon Michael Dogali, in which patients with Parkinsonism who had small pieces of their brains removed showed significant improvement. One researcher on the experiment, neurologist Enrico Fazzini, said that outcome perhaps indicated that the improvement noted in the Denver and Yale patients was caused not by fetal cells but by the cuts themselves, as Landau has hypothesized. It seems that despite its claims to the contrary, the *L.A. Times* will need more proof.

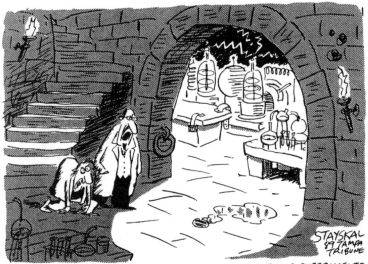

"THE GOVERNMENT STILL WON'T FUND OUR FETAL TISSUE EXPERIMENTS IGOR... I THINK THEY'RE LIVING IN THE DARK AGES!"

Landau says that one means by which fetal cell transplants could conceivably work would be by acting as a pump, as with diabetes patients. "But the cells injected have to be able to react to blood sugar the way normal cells do," and this could be problematic. "On the other hand, maybe they wouldn't regulate but could serve as reservoir. But then why not just put a slow-leaking bottle of levadopa into the brain?" (In fact, pocket-sized insulin pumps for diabetics will soon be in general use.) "The irreversible tragedy is the death and damage to many patients and their families produced by the extravagance of the transplantation fad," he said.

At the 1989 annual meeting of the American Association of Neurological Surgeons in Washington, D.C., as the *Journal of the American Medical Association* (*JAMA*) put it, "The consensus [was] that while [grafting] is still promising, particularly when fetal brain tissue is grafted, new side effects are continuing to emerge." Specifically noted was the breaking of the blood-brain barrier that persisted for several months after surgery in six patients. Such breaches can prove fatal.

Rejected Tissue

In general, fetal neural cells are less likely to cause rejection than adult tissue from another person. They often fail to cause significant immune responses when implanted in rodents and apes, and have been used in successful human operations without immune suppression. However, animal studies comparing the immunogenicity of fetal pancreas with adult pancreas cells show that the fetal tissue can be as immune-incompatible, if not more so, than adult tissue. Fetal liver cells have also prompted immune responses.

Researcher George Allen, of the Vanderbilt University Medical School, head of the most experienced American group in brain graft therapy, says: "Putting aside the practical and ethical problems of getting donor tissue . . . there is the issue of graft rejection. We've seen signs of rejection in some experimental animals, and we don't know what this would mean in functional terms in humans. Presumably, long-term immunosuppression would be necessary." He adds: "We don't know what fetal tissue would do over a period of many years. There's a possibility it could grow and become an invasive tumor."

"Why," asks Father Robert Barry, a bioethicist at the University of Illinois, "should these patients be put into a life-threatening condition in order to alleviate one that is only debilitating?". . .

Transplant opponents argue that there is no reason to portray providing therapy for Parkinson's disease patients or patients of other diseases as an either-or situation: either fetal cell transplants will help them or nothing will. Indeed, they say, all this fuss is a distraction from therapies that may prove cheaper, less painful, and more permanent, with the bonus that they completely bypass the touchy ethical issues. There are many alternative therapies either just around the corner or already being tried out.

It is difficult to predict developments for Parkinson's and other brain disorders because pharmaceutical and biotechnical companies guard their research very closely, and because the hype that has pervaded the fetal cell transplant area is common to all research science. But one drug recently put into use, Deprenyl, substantially slows the rate of neurodegeneration in Parkinsonian patients, according to a *Science* article by neurologists James Tetrud and William Langston. Deprenyl inhibits monoamine oxidase, a substance present in many different body cells and one that breaks down dopamine. "The magnitude of the effect is much greater than we could have hoped for," says Langston. "I suspect that very soon Deprenyl will find a place in the early treatment of Parkinson's disease.

In *Science*, two scientists reported their discovery that mouse brain tissue, when stimulated by NGF in a laboratory dish, has the capacity to produce new nerve cells. This discovery challenges the traditional view that the brain cells of post-natal mammals cannot regenerate. The scientists have yet to try to reproduce these results in living mice, but—considering that the cells in question are from the same part of the brain affected by Parkinson's, Huntington's, and other diseases; that a transplant would come from the person himself, thus negating the possibility of rejection; and that the cells would be adult ones—the ramifications would be tremendous.

This report was followed by one describing an almost complete reversal of Parkinsonism symptoms that had been induced in monkeys. The monkeys were injected with a substance derived from cow brains. Whether it will work in humans with actual Parkinson's disease remains to be seen, but the substance has already been used on humans with spinal cord injuries, with significant improvement shown.

Surpassed by Other Technology

However effective fetal cell transplantation turns out to be, it could well be surpassed by other technology before it comes to fruition, rather like the astronaut in the "Twilight Zone" television series who returns from a forty-year round-trip visit to a distant planet only to find that he has wasted half his life because faster ships have been developed since he left and have beaten him back to earth. At worst, fetal cell transplants may be the equivalent of the Jarvik-7—little more than an instrument of torture for the brave souls who assume guinea pig status for it. Given the lack of good animal data, the scarcity of medical research funds in general, and not least of all the repugnancy that much of society has toward using human tissue that was not consensually given, . . . fetal tissue research [should be abandoned].

"We had fought this disease for eleven years and finally tried something experimental. . . . [The consequence] was one big hallelujah chorus."

Fetal Tissue Research Offers Hope to Disease Victims

Jeff Goldberg and Anne Hollister

In the February 1992 edition of *Life* magazine, writer Jeff Goldberg, assisted by reporter Anne Hollister, told the story of Terri and Guy Walden, who had two children born with Hurler's syndrome, a debilitating and ultimately fatal genetic disease. Offered a chance to save their third, as yet unborn, Hurler's child, the Waldens faced a crisis of conscience. Guy Walden is a Baptist minister and neither he nor his wife believe in abortion, yet their child's chance to live would depend on the liver tissue of an aborted fetus. The Waldens, like many others, ultimately decided that fetal tissue offers a chance to bring something good out of what they perceive as the immoral act of abortion. After their experience, the Waldens testified before Congress in an effort to rescind the rules prohibiting the use of tissues from aborted fetuses.

As you read, consider the following questions:

1. List two factors, besides the fate of their unborn son, that helped the Waldens decide to allow the use of fetal tissue.
2. The Waldens believed using the tissues of aborted fetuses allowed something good to come out of an immoral act, and that, in fact, to waste the tissue would be wrong. Do you agree? Explain.

Excerpts of "Who Gets to Play God?" by Jeff Goldberg and Anne Hollister, *Life*, February 1992. Reprinted with permission.

Every morning, day after day, Terri and Guy Walden would wake up with the same anxiety and head for their daughter Angie's room. They'd turn the knob, slowly, in dread, facing the worst fear parents can know. Their firstborn, Jason, had died in his sleep at the age of eight of Hurler's syndrome, a rare genetic disease. Seven-year-old Angie also had Hurler's, and they knew she, too, would soon be dead. Their two other children, Hannah and John, do not have the disease. During the spring of 1990, as Angie's decline overwhelmed the Waldens, Terri became pregnant again. Testing revealed that the child growing inside her had Hurler's.

The vast majority of American parents-to-be choose abortion when faced with test results showing a serious genetic disorder. The Waldens, however, do not condone abortion under any circumstances. They are southern Baptists who served as missionaries in the Amazon jungles, and Guy is pastor of the evangelical Broadway Baptist Temple in Houston. "Abortion violates God's law; it's a wrongful death," Guy says. It seemed that only a miracle could save their unborn child from deformity and certain death, yet a miracle was at hand. Ironically, it was a miracle that, because of their beliefs, the Waldens might not be able to accept.

A Hurler's specialist in Minnesota put the couple in touch with two medical researchers, physiologist Esmail Zanjani and obstetrician Nathan Slotnick. Experimenting on sheep and monkeys, they had developed a technique that might allow healthy cells from an aborted fetus to be transplanted into a living fetus before it was born. The technique had never been tried on humans, but Zanjani and Slotnick hoped fetal liver cells—injected into the Waldens' unborn child—would find their way to bone marrow, where they might grow and eventually produce a critical enzyme. Without the enzyme, fats and sugars clump together like deposits of Krazy Glue, wreaking havoc in every tissue and organ of the body. The Waldens knew the symptoms well—Angie's features were wrinkled and wizened into a cruel parody of old age; she could no longer walk, and she had to sleep in an oxygen tent. . . .

Crisis of Conscience

For the overjoyed Waldens, opportunity brought crisis: How could they live with the fact that the tissue being used to save their child's life would come from an aborted fetus? With only three weeks to decide what to do—the procedure had to be done before Terri's 18th week of pregnancy—the Waldens turned to friends, other pastors and lawyers for advice. They were stunned by the lack of support. Members of Broadway Baptist Temple, for example, often greeted the news with stares. "They

130

all saw it in terms of the abortion issue, and all the people we know are against it. So each just said, 'I wouldn't want to be in your shoes. I wouldn't want to make that decision,'" Terri remembers.

Slotnick flew in from Sacramento to talk to them. "He knew that parents in our situation are left with only two choices, both negative," Guy Walden says. "One, to abort the baby, which we are very opposed to, and two, to watch the child die. He wanted to offer parents like us a positive alternative. If this worked, it would significantly aid research in treating many rare genetic diseases. We are pro-life. We wanted to help the living."

Struggling to reason their way through flesh-and-blood realities, the Waldens began to think that fetal tissue should be treated like the donated kidneys, hearts and bone marrow that are used to save thousands of lives each year. "Abortion and fetal tissue transplants are two separate issues," Guy says. "We're very much opposed to abortion, but right now it's legal, and to let the tissue from these babies rot in the trash means letting children die who might be saved. We aren't talking about ideology here, we're talking about hope."

Slotnick offered them another salve for their consciences: Fetal tissue transplants might actually reduce the number of abortions. Thousands of fetuses are aborted every year because serious genetic diseases have been detected. Many of those diseases might be reversed by transplants like the one proposed for the Walden fetus.

Biblical Support Found

Finally, the Waldens found what they really had to have—passages in the Bible they could interpret as proof that God was on their side. "There's a verse in Genesis about how God took one of Adam's ribs and made Eve, so it seemed clear enough that God was not against tissue transplants," Guy says. And in Proverbs, he read: "Trust in the Lord with all thine heart; and lean not unto thine own understanding." Guy took that to mean "if God did not want us to do this, he would stop it by not allowing it to go through."

The Waldens set a date for the operation: May 23, 1990. . . .

For months after the transplant, Terri and Guy Walden lived in suspense, not knowing if the procedure had worked or failed. Though they were trying to go about their lives with some order and reason, 1990 was an incredibly difficult year. In February Terri discovered she was pregnant, in March that the child would have Hurler's disease, in April that she would be accepted for the experiment.

Four months after the transplant, in September, Terri was driving Angie, Hannah and John to catch her husband's evening service at the little brick church in the poor section of Houston called Broadway. "I looked in the rearview mirror and Angie was gone, slumped over in her seat. Just a half hour earlier she was playing." Terri ran two red lights racing for the hospital. Police interrupted Guy's service, and he rushed to the hospital. It was hopeless. Angie was already dead.

Pro-Life Miracles

For those of us facing the nightmare of advanced Parkinsonism—a lethal blend of rigidity, tremor and motor dysfunction, eventually robbing the ability to walk, eat, talk, even move—this development is a dream come true.

And more good news will follow: Fetal tissue transplants appear to be reversing diabetes symptoms, and may be a possible therapy for many other chronic degenerative conditions. . . .

Since abortion is wrong, [some reason,] no benefit should result, even if it would save a life. But punishing me for another's moral choice—a choice that will be made anyway—doesn't even out the equation. It just harms more people. . . .

Shouldn't we encourage such miracles? How can it be "pro-life" to stop them?

Joan Samuelson Corbett, *Los Angeles Times*, September 19, 1990.

In October Terri and Guy traveled to Sacramento, where Slotnick induced delivery. Nathan Adam Walden (named for Slotnick) remained in the hospital until a week before Christmas. He showed indications the graft was taking hold but no signs whatsoever that it was producing the essential enzyme. The Waldens, though, sensed something was happening. "All Hurler's children have a constant runny nose and are unable to raise their hands above their heads, but Nathan didn't show either of those," Terri says.

Hallelujah Chorus

However, months went by and Nathan continued to test negative for the enzyme. When the Waldens testified before the Senate, they had little reason to believe he would make it. Still, they fought for the right of others to try the same experiment. Low on hope, they decided after six months of negative tests to try a bone marrow transplant on Nathan, using marrow from one of his siblings. The operation itself, which is life-threatening and very expensive, was unlikely to be completely successful. The Waldens would have to stay in Minnesota, where the operation would be performed, for three months while Nathan recovered. "We were packing to go when we got the call," Terri says. It was Slotnick, who had asked to do a final round of tests. The transplant had worked—enough enzyme was showing up to indicate that Nathan had indeed developed a new source of blood cells.

"You can't describe it," Guy says. "We had fought this disease for eleven years and finally tried something experimental. Then apparently it didn't work. Our hopes were dashed. Then that call came. All of a sudden it felt like life had been worth it. It was one big hallelujah chorus."

Nathan's future is still up in the air. Zanjani says that "despite the presence of the enzyme, we really don't know if this is going to be ultimately therapeutic. It is a good sign, and we have established that this can be done safely without any adverse effect on the baby and that even in this very first try there is a degree of success. It would be fantastic if this was sufficient to prevent the baby from having any further deterioration."

In the meantime, Nathan's body is continuing to produce increased amounts of the enzyme and he has passed into the low-normal range of enzyme levels. Though the results may be less than perfect, for Guy Walden it is "nothing short of a miracle."

"None of this has been easy," says Terri, who is pregnant again. The Waldens do not believe in birth control. Terri's physicians tell her this baby will be fine, but if it is not, she insists, "I would have the transplant again. We've seen the results. It works."

> "A fetus, electively aborted, is an innocent, developing human being that has been offered up as a living sacrifice to propitiate some lesser god of expediency."

Fetal Tissue Research Is Immoral

Sharon Fish

Sharon Fish, a nurse and the author of *Alzheimer's: Caring for Your Loved One, Caring for Yourself*, is the daughter of an Alzheimer's victim. Recent biomedical research has offered promise that the injection of fetal brain tissue can alleviate or devastating disease of mind and body. Yet Fish is adamantly against the use of such tissue, even to save the life of her mother and other disease victims. No good can come out of the evil act of harvesting the tissue of living human beings murdered by abortion, she asserts.

As you read, consider the following questions:

1. Fish says the logic that seeks to justify fetal tissue use is "twisted, tangled, and flawed." What examples of illogic does she point out?
2. On what basis does Fish believe it is nobler to suffer a fatal or debilitating disease than to seek a cure through the use of fetal tissue?

Sharon Fish, "The Scandal of Fetal-Tissue Research," *Christianity Today*, November 19, 1990. Reprinted with permission.

"If you allowed yourselves to think of God, you wouldn't allow yourselves to be degraded by pleasant vices. You'd have a reason for bearing things patiently, for doing things with courage. I've seen it with the Indians."

"I'm sure you have," said Mustapha Mond. "But then we aren't Indians. There isn't any need for a civilized man to bear anything that's seriously unpleasant."

Aldous Huxley, Brave New World

There are many unpleasant, even savage, diseases that wreak havoc in the lives of both loved ones and those who love. I know about this havoc firsthand: My mother has Alzheimer's disease.

Alzheimer's is a chronic, irreversible brain disorder, or dementia. Its chief characteristics are senile plaques of amyloid protein laid down between nerve cells, inhibiting message transmission. Microscopic fibers, resembling twisted, tangled threads of yarn, also cluster in brain cell nuclei, mixing up the mind, obliterating memory.

The biomedical community says human fetal-tissue research and transplantation (HFTRT) offers hope—if not for my mother, perhaps for me should my own memory start slipping down the slope toward that abyss.

But that held-out hope demands a terrible, unbearable cost. The price tag is innocent lives destroyed by even crueler acts of savagery than the ravages of a dementia: the savagery of elective, on-demand abortion.

Twisted Logic

The logic seeking to justify HFTRT using deliberately aborted fetuses is as twisted as the neurofibrillary tangles inside my mother's mind: twisted, tangled, and flawed.

The principal argument in favor of a full-speed-ahead approach is that abortion and HFTRT are separate and distinct issues. You can hate the one yet embrace the other. Even if you grant that elective abortion is an essentially evil act, it is argued that salvaging and using the fetal remains for good purposes does *not* connote complicity with the abortion itself.

The analogy frequently used is that of transplantation with organs derived from victims of homicide. If it is ethical to transplant those organs made available through a violent, illegal act, why not use fetal tissue from an albeit violent, but still legal act?

No complicity? Nonsense!

There is a general consensus among ethicists and researchers alike that a new "feel better" philosophy will result for both fetal donors and those who perform elective abortions if that fetus can be used to benefit humankind. Researchers and those receiving fetal tissue are not simply passive beneficiaries. They are, rather, actively providing opportunities to assuage both individual and collective guilt.

The same thing as an organ transplant? Absurd!

A fetus is not a heart or a liver, a kidney or a cornea. A fetus, electively aborted, is an innocent, developing human being that has been offered up as a living sacrifice to propitiate some lesser god of expediency, whose chief aim seems to be to rid us of anything (or anyone) that might make our lives unpleasant—even for a short a time as nine months.

Ends Contradicted by Means

It is clear enough: the ends are contradicted by the means. Taking innocent human lives in order to save other human lives undermines a basic principle of the moral code that sustains our society and the legal code that regulates our common life. . . . To refer to fetal tissue as if it were mere tissue disembedded from its human provenance, or to speak of finding it in a trash can as if magically transported from we-know-not-where, evades the morally obvious. Of course, fetal tissue is human tissue—not even *Roe v. Wade* denies that. This tissue was once part of a developing life that has been destroyed and dispatched. Harvesting that tissue in order to save or sustain another, wanted human life cannot redeem the taking of life in the first place (drawing good out of evil). For that reason after World War II the scientific community chose to forego whatever knowledge might derive from Nazi medical experiments.

Commonweal, June 19, 1992.

The procurement and use of this human fetal tissue to enhance or elongate the life of another human being is *not* a simple salvage operation. It is, purely and simply, cannibalism.

The parent of a child gunned down by a homicidal maniac or whose life has otherwise been extinguished by illness or accident, *does* have the right to choose what to do with all or parts of their loved one's body. The parent of a child electively aborted does *not* have that right. The issue of consent is no longer moot.

Having relegated the unborn to the status of nonhuman or prehuman, to give consent for the fetal remains following an elective abortion would imply the fetus was human after all. If this is the case, the parent is not simply a stranger who has abrogated rights as a result of the abortion, but is, in fact, the one responsible for the child's death. Those who compare fetal-tissue transplantation to organ transplantation should take time to carry out their analogy to its logical conclusion.

"If you allow yourselves to think of God . . . you'd have a reason for bearing things patiently, for doing things with courage," said John Savage in Huxley's *Brave New World*. Patience and courage are two virtues sadly needed, in the research laboratories today that are bent on justifying the morality of fetal-tissue research and transplantations.

Patience and Courage

Patience is needed to wait: to wait for fetal tissue spontaneously or nonelectively aborted that doesn't bear the taint of sin. Patience is needed to pursue other, perhaps related, but ethically neutral avenues of inquiry.

Courage is needed, too. To seek to justify HFTRT by imbuing deliberately induced abortions with redeeming social value is the ultimate act of cowardice. The fact that justification is thought to be needed at all tells a tale. Morally righteous acts need no justification. So courage is needed to resist the vocal lobbyists representing sufferers of diseases like Alzheimer's, Parkinson's, juvenile diabetes, and AIDS, and to urge them to wait for treatments and cures that offer hope but also a peace of conscience for all concerned.

The supreme act of courage would be for researchers and ethicists alike just to say "no more" to certain avenues of inquiry. That slippery slope of ethical decision making needs fewer one-way streets and more roadblocks—not as obstacles to go around or over, but as places for rest, re-evaluation, and retreat. There is a desperate need for bio-medical science to re-evaluate its understanding of suffering in light of the sovereignty of God. To do so may mean rewriting certain scripts and a giving up of certain powers. That, too, will be an act of courage, and for many people unaccustomed to restraint, a seriously unpleasant thought.

> *"It is evident that experimentation on aborted children has less to do with helping sick people than with justifying the abortion industry."*

The Use of Fetal Tissue Would Encourage Abortion

Rebecca Ryskind

Rebecca Ryskind is an antiabortion lobbyist in Washington, D.C. In the following viewpoint, she expresses her belief that allowing the use of fetal tissue in medical research will ultimately ennoble abortion, an act she believes is morally indefensible.

As you read, consider the following questions:

1. In what way might the use of fetal tissue cause abortion to be viewed as a noble act, according to the author?
2. Why does Ryskind believe government funded fetal tissue research will increase the number of abortions?
3. Why does Ryskind believe the potential good that may come from fetal tissue research does not justify such research?

Condensed from Rebecca Ryskind, "Fatal Tissue," *Human Life Review*, Summer 1992. Reprinted with permission.

The question of whether the federal government ought to fund research on aborted children has recurred periodically since 1975, when an "Ethical Advisory Board" at the Department of Health, Education and Welfare approved experimentation on aborted—but still living—fetuses. Public outcry when the nature of such experiments was revealed brought a temporary end to the research, not only because of its grisly character, but also because the people recognized no clear purpose in experiments such as severing the heads from aborted babies and maintaining their brains alive.

But fetal tissue research is no longer on the grotesque fringe of science. Some researchers have suggested that fetal tissue—particularly fetal brain tissue—may be spectacularly regenerative and adaptable, and hence suitable for transplant into victims of diabetes, Parkinson's and Alzheimer's disease for near-miraculous cures. This unsubstantiated promise of relief for millions of sufferers has brought fetal research to the forefront of the abortion battle. . . .

Justifying the Abortion Industry

When the facts of the case are laid out, it is evident that experimentation on aborted children has less to do with helping sick people than with justifying the abortion industry. The effect will not, of course, be immediate, and therein lies part of the problem. People who should know better have been persuaded that "safeguards" (e.g., preventing the aborting mother from specifying the recipient of her baby's tissue) will prevent any abuse. But opponents point out that once the barrier between abortion and government funding is penetrated, it can be only a matter of time before the supposed safeguards are shunted aside. As Georgetown University Professor Daniel Robinson—a member of the 1988 NIH [National Institutes of Health] panel on fetal tissue transplantation—put it one evening on CNN's *Crossfire*, we can establish safeguards in 1992, but ". . . if it turned out that a significant public health problem could be addressed by taking down that so-called impenetrable wall, how long do you think it would be before some progressive and right-thinking Congressman" would move to strike down the barriers? . . . Abortion proponents can afford to be generous with "safeguards" because they know that safeguards never last long. They deride the notion of a slippery slope even as they take advantage of it in achieving their ends in Congress.

Some tactical ground may have been ceded to the abortionists when the Bush Administration adopted as its chief argument against the bill the possibility that potential good coming from research would encourage women to have abortions. This triggered angry complaints from feminist groups that the White

House was "patronizing" women, suggesting they choose to have abortions lightly. But no one has suggested that fetal tissue research will cause women to become cavalier about abortion; the issue is that abortion itself may become ennobled. As Professor Robinson put it, "To do something that will save other human lives is not to do something cavalier." Again, fetal tissue experimentation is only the first step. Once it is tolerated it will be embraced. Once embraced, what then? How long before we have an unregulated "fetus industry" in which the organs of unborn babies are bought and sold as commonly as pints of blood? . . .

Babies as Biological Raw Material

Treating unborn babies as a kind of medical cornucopia would be unwise in any circumstance. . . .

It is no accident that abortion supporters combine one highly questionable assumption—that fetal tissue therapy will work—with a second even more dubious proposition—that the federal government by statute can establish (or, for that matter, disestablish) fundamental rights. Both are part of a larger agenda of maintaining abortion on demand. . . .

Fetal tissue transplants are dubious science, ethically bankrupt and an open invitation to treat the unborn as so much biological raw material. They should be vigorously opposed.

Dave Andrusko, *Priorities*, Summer 1992.

The *New York Times* once called the comparison between abortion and the Holocaust "obscene." Contemporary researchers bridle at any analogy between themselves and Nazi scientists. The fact remains that, as Joseph Sobran noted (in a column titled "The Angel of Choice"), the Nazi researchers shared the premises of some of those who think they are exactly the opposite of Nazis. Writing of Dr. Joseph Mengele, the Nazi "angel of death" who spent the latter years of his life working as an abortionist in Argentina, Sobran says:

He saw himself as a progressive, and he was right. He had liberated himself from stifling moral traditions, and he was in the vanguard of change, seeking new scientific answers through experimentation. He shared the Darwinian materialism of his time, which is still our time, even if the Nazi wing has gone a little out of fashion. Abortion, fetal experimentation, surrogate motherhood, genetic engineering—he would have been right at home with these new developments. In fact, he could fairly consider himself a pioneer, a casualty of progress who was ahead of his time.

The "murderous science" of the Nazis didn't begin with Hitler and it didn't begin overnight. Eugenics programs—always begun in the name of high humanitarian principles—were well established during the Weimar Republic. Germany didn't accidentally wake up evil one morning; the German people simply got slowly accustomed to breaking down the safeguards separating science from atrocity.

"Squandering" Good Material

The late Dr. Leo Alexander, a consultant at the Nuremberg trials once interviewed a Nazi doctor who defended his experimentation on the carefully-removed brains of 100 Holocaust victims. *He* was not a murderer, he argued, because *he* had not marked the victims for death. But it would have been a shame to squander "such wonderful material!" It would have been a pity not to get something good for humanity from their deaths!

Is that not the precise argument of those who ask with respect to fetal tissue experimentation: "Why not"? Wouldn't it be a pity not to get something good for humanity from the babies marked for death in any case? With all due respect to Senator Thurmond, when he asked from the Senate floor, "If this is going to help humanity, why not do it? What could be the objection to it?" was he not rejecting the world's collective verdict at Nuremberg? The world indeed decided at Nuremberg that it had numerous objections—chief among them the judgment that "progress" erected over the graves of the innocent is not worth achieving.

Fascination and Danger

Not that progress doesn't have its attractions. In her best-selling novel, *The Witching Hour*, Anne Rice explores the fascination and danger of fetal research from a scientist's point of view:

"I saw it in the incubator, this little fetus. Do you know what he called it? He called it the abortus. . . . and this thing had been sustained, alive," she said, "from a four-month abortion, and you know he was developing means of live support for even younger fetuses. He was talking of breeding embryos in test tubes and never returning them to the womb at all, but all of this to harvest organs. You should have heard his arguments, that the fetus was playing a vital role in the human life chain, could you believe it, and I'll tell you the horrible part, the really horrible part, it was that it was utterly fascinating, and I loved it. I saw the potential uses he was describing. I knew it would be possible some day to create new and undamaged brains for coma victims. Oh, God, you know all the things that could be done, the things that I, given my talent, could have done!"

He nodded. "I can see it," he said softly, "I can see the horror of it and I can see the lure."

Is the real creed of our Science that what we can do, we must do? There is no question but that "progress"—no matter how achieved—can be enticing. But it is equally clear that by funding research on aborted babies, even under supposedly well-controlled circumstances, our Congress will be opening Pandora's Box. As Daniel Robinson noted (citing Hegel) in his debate on *Crossfire*: "What the state permits, it encourages."

"It [is] 'highly unlikely,' even farfetched, that a woman would choose abortion because she knows the fetal remains will be used in a transplant."

The Use of Fetal Tissue Would Not Encourage Abortion

The American Jewish Congress Bio-Ethics Task Force

The American Jewish Congress, a national organization focusing on the arts and other aspects of Jewish life and culture, was one of several organizations that offered testimony to the congressional committee that determined whether to allow federal funding to resume for fetal tissue research. The AJC's Bio-Ethics Task Force asserted that allowing such research would not encourage abortions, that abortion is, in any case, a personal decision for a woman, and that fetal tissue research promises much benefit to humanity. The task force recommended that Congress rescind the moratorium on federal funding, which it later did.

As you read, consider the following questions:

1. What factors led the task force to believe that allowing fetal tissue research would not encourage more abortions?
2. What position does the task force take on deliberately conceiving a donor fetus?
3. Why does the task force consider the Holocaust analogy, popular with those opposed to fetal tissue research, inapt?

From the April 15, 1991, statement by the American Jewish Congress Bio-Ethics Task Force submitted to the U.S. House of Representatives Committee on Energy and Commerce, Subcommittee on Health and the Environment.

143

The [American Jewish Congress Bio-Ethics] Task Force does not believe that use of fetal tissue for transplant research will either encourage individual women to have abortions, legitimize abortion in society generally, "confer" dignity or prestige on abortion practitioners or provide a financial incentive to increase abortions.

Research shows that most women choose to abort for a number of reasons, all weighty, and all involving each woman's unique and very personal circumstances. Among those reasons are her economic, marital and family situation and her own assessment of her ability to fulfill the lifetime commitment of concern and care which motherhood demands. Like the NIH [National Institutes of Health] Panel majority, the Task Force therefore believes it "highly unlikely," even farfetched, that a woman would choose abortion because she knows the fetal remains will be used in a transplant procedure for an anonymous other individual or even that the decision of an ambivalent woman would be tipped in favor of an abortion because she knew the fetal remains might be used for that purpose. Physicians and others who work closely with women who make the decision to abort have stated that these views attribute unwarranted weight to secondary considerations and show a basic misunderstanding of the nature of the principal reasons women choose to abort.

Prohibiting the sale or purchase of fetal tissue will eliminate any significant financial incentive to procure or encourage abortion. Nor is it likely that allowing reimbursement of costs will enhance abortion clinic revenues; that argument is premised on speculation that transplantation therapy will be so enormously successful, demand for fetal tissue will exceed supply. At best, that is many years away, and it is time enough to deal with that problem when and if it materializes. Furthermore, researchers are also working on developing cultured cells that would minimize the need for fetal tissue in the future.

Little Benefit to Intra-Family Donations

The argument based on the hypothetical claim that women will deliberately conceive and abort to obtain fetal remains to aid a family member must be distinguished from the argument that a woman's decision to abort, admittedly made for other more personal reasons, will be influenced by the fact that the fetal remains might possibly aid some anonymous others.

The Task Force, as indicated, finds the latter situation to be speculative in the extreme. The issue of intra-family donations is also hypothetical. There is no medical evidence that intra-family donations are preferable or even medically indicated. The transplantation of purified fetal cells does not require tissue matching as is necessary with bone marrow transplants. In fact, with certain genetically transmitted diseases, such as Type I diabetes, they may even be contraindicated since they increase the risk of reappearance of the disease.

How Transplants Might Be Used

Fetal tissue type	Could possibly treat:
Liver and Thymus	Leukemia Aplastic anemia Inherited metabolic disorders Radiation injuries Severe Combined Immune Deficiency
Pancreas	Diabetes

Neural tissue	Vision impairment
	Spinal-cord injuries
	Memory deficits
	
	Degenerative diseases including:
	  Huntington's chorea
	  Alzheimer's
	  Parkinson's

Source: *Time*, April 6, 1992.

It is possible, if not likely, that medical research may develop to the point that intra-family donations are not only medically indicated but lifesaving. In that event, a society which currently permits a mother or father or a twin sibling or anyone to possibly shorten their lifespan by donating a kidney might well permit a mother to conceive and abort a fetus to save an existing dying child or similar close relative.

Deliberate Donor Conception Is a Personal Decision

Deliberately conceiving to abort for altruistic reasons, whether to aid an anonymous sufferer or a particular family member, is subject to the ethical objection that one may be treating a potential human as a means to an end. However, a decision to conceive and abort to aid another is intensely personal and reflects the religious and ethical values of the woman making this decision. As a general rule women should not be encouraged or persuaded to conceive and abort to aid another. Nevertheless, the Task Force recognizes the extremely strong and ethically appropriate bonds of love and concern which link members of the nuclear family. In light of these bonds, the Task Force believes it would be unrealistic and morally unsound, at this juncture, to foreclose for all time a donation of fetal tissue obtained specifically to aid a family member when necessary to spare life or alleviate very severe suffering, if the abortion takes place before the fetus develops neurological or cognitive capacity and cannot experience pain.

However, because there is no current scientific evidence that intra-family donations are presently or ever will be therapeutic, a decision on this difficult ethical issue can be postponed to some future time. In the meantime, alternative therapies that do not involve fetal tissue may become available. At any rate, the knowledge that difficult ethical dilemmas lie ahead should not serve as an ethical argument in opposition to funding promising research now.

Safeguards Would Prevent Dignity of Fetus

In the meantime, the Task Force shares the NIH's Panel's view—adopted by even some opponents of abortion serving on that body—that with appropriate safeguards the decision to abort can be separated from the subsequent research use of fetal tissue. These safeguards assure that neither the researchers nor the recipient of the tissue would have any role in inducing or encouraging the abortion, and that a woman's decision making would be insulated from any concerns about subsequent use of the fetal tissue for transplant research and therapy. The Task Force also believes that these safeguards protect the dignity of the fetus and ensure that the woman's health remains the paramount concern.

Among the specific safeguards the NIH panel urged, and that the AJCongress Task Force generally recommends and supports, are:

1. The decision to terminate a pregnancy and the procedures of abortion should be kept independent from the retrieval and use of fetal tissue.

2. Payments and other forms of remuneration and compensation associated with the procurement of fetal tissue should be prohibited, except payment for reasonable expenses occasioned by the actual retrieval, storage, preparation, and transportation of the tissue.

3. The decision and consent to abort must precede discussion of the possible use of the fetal tissue and any request for such consent as might be required for that use.

4. The timing and method of abortion should not be influenced by the potential uses of fetal tissue for transplantation or medical research.

5. Fetal tissue from induced abortions should not be used in medical research without the prior consent of the pregnant woman.

6. The consent should be obtained in compliance with State law and with the Uniform Anatomical Gift Act.

The transplantation of organs either from a live donor or from a cadaver is now considered morally acceptable, even morally commendable, if the donor or the donor's proxy has given informed and uncoerced consent. One of the thorniest problems in the fetal tissue area centers on who ethically can give consent to use fetal tissue when the fetus has been deliberately aborted.

Under UAGA, either parent can "donate" fetal remains provided the other parent does not object. Some theorists, however, have questioned whether a parent who has collaborated in the destruction of a fetus can morally act as the fetus' proxy. These theorists view proxy donations as premised on the idea that one who cares for another, like a parent for a child, will act in that person's interest even after death. But if the parent has acted as the agent of death, he or she has abandoned any interest in the child's care and cannot act as its protective proxy.

Under this view, if there is no one who can act as the protective proxy, then fetal remains cannot ethically be confiscated without demeaning the dignity of the fetus in a way society has considered ethically unacceptable for other cadavers. As Dr. Kathleen Nolan of the Hastings Center writes:

> To make fetuses the harbingers of a move toward routine salvage as a basic mode of cadaveric treatment would . . . manifest a harsh but fairly consistent historical practice of looking first to society's outcasts when new necrogenous materials (such as autopsy specimens) are needed.

According to Professor John Robertson, however, the entire notion of protective proxy is misguided since deceased persons and fetuses no longer have interests that can be protected by proxy. Rather, it is the interests of the next-of-kin that underlie laws on organ donations and a woman who has chosen to abort still has an interest and may deeply care how the product of her body is disposed. She, therefore, is entitled to have her wishes, including her consent to donate, honored by law.

The AJCongress Bio-Ethics Task Force agrees with this analysis. Despite the decision to abort, a pregnant woman retains a special connection with the fetus that gives her a legitimate interest in the disposal of its remains. Indeed, the Task Force believes that this connection is so vital, maternal consent should be *required* before fetal tissue is used in medical procedures.

The Question of Complicity

Another source of the opposition to fetal tissue research by those who view abortion as morally objectionable focuses on the moral complicity of scientists who use the fetus derived from an abortion, and of society if it participates in that use by permitting, even funding, this type of research or procedures. These opponents maintain that medical research with fetal remains cannot be disassociated from the abortion and that procedures designed to insulate the researcher from the abortion process simply ignore the inevitable link between those who take advantage of an immoral act and the underlying act itself.

Some, including the dissenters on the NIH Panel, have analogized the moral complicity of fetal tissue researchers, and the government if it funds the research, with the moral complicity of Nazi doctors who engaged in medical experimentation on live prisoners or on the cadavers or organs of murdered prisoners. They point out that many of these doctors claimed that they had nothing to do with supplying the bodies, and, since the prisoners were invariably executed anyway, they were ethically permitted to conduct experiments that might produce some good from the prisoners' deaths. This claim, the argument goes, like similar claims made by fetal tissue researchers, fails to recognize moral complicity after the fact.

The Bio-Ethics Task Force considers abortion to be morally acceptable and therefore does not consider it to be morally objectionable to participate directly or indirectly in the procedure. The Holocaust analogy, therefore, is simply inapt. An abortion on a non-sentient, non-cognitive fetus of rudimentary development is a far cry from the torture of unconsenting, fully developed human beings who can feel apprehension and pain. The enormity of the horror and misery associated with the Nazi experiments makes it understandable that society would want to distance itself from these experiments and that Jewish and other scientists should suggest that use of data derived from these grisly experiments should be banned for fear of giving the experiments legitimacy or encouraging future societies to replicate them.

An Ethical Procedure

Because the Task Force does not find abortion to be in any comparable to the Nazis' activities it believes such distancing is not necessary and use of fetal remains from abortions to save lives is permissible and ethically appropriate.

Even, however, if one accepts the view that abortion is an immoral act, one need not reject the fruits of abortion to save lives for fear of implying approval of and becoming an accomplice to the abortion act after the fact. The doctor who participates in or the patient who enjoys the benefit from the transplantation of an organ obtained from a homicide victim is not complicit in the homicide that made the organ available. Both the recipients of the fetal remains derived from an abortion in which they did not participate, and the researchers using those remains, are morally innocent of complicity in the abortion. Thus, if, as we urge, the decision to donate fetal tissue and the procurement of the tissue are separated from the subsequent use of the tissue, that use is not, by itself, in any way morally problematic.

Research with fetal tissue, particularly if it leads to successful transplantation, also raises concern over whether pregnant women will be exploited by a medical system that places the need for fetal tissue over the welfare of women. Some question whether the safety of the abortion procedure might be compromised by the desire to make optimal use of the fetal tissue. Others believe that women of lower socio-economic classes will become the most frequent donors of fetal tissue and that educational efforts designed to decrease the number of unwanted pregnancies among the poor will be thwarted by an increasing need for fetal tissue. Still others see fetal tissue research as an aspect of the commodification of a woman's body and fear that women, who are ingrained with the idea that their role is to nurture, will consider the "harvesting" of their tissue for the good of others as furthering this role.

Good Outweighs Ethical Problems

The Bio-Ethics Task Force, while understanding the basis for these concerns, believes that they too are so speculative they are outweighted by the enormous good that may come from fetal tissue research. There is unanimity concerning the ethical proposition that the safety of the pregnant woman is of paramount importance. At the present time, researchers generally prefer fetal tissue derived from first trimester abortions. The needs of medical research, therefore, now coincide with medical standards on the safest timing and method of abortion. Moreover, current protocols for privately funded research, as well as existing medical ethics, demand that the woman's health be accorded the utmost concern. For example, The American College of Obstetricians and Gynecologists mandates that research concerns not "affect advice about the decision to have an abortion, its timing, or the method employed to induce the abortion." The NIH Panel made a similar recommendation and AJCongress Task Force concurs.

The Task Force also believes that banning the commercial exploitation of fetal tissue will eliminate any incentive for the poor to become pregnant in order to donate fetal remains. The advent of cadaver organ transplantation has not led to any exploitation of the poor or to any compromise in the terminal care of potential organ donors. Finally, the possibility that society will redirect efforts away from family planning is simply too unlikely to justify a ban on research that could be of incalculable value.

Periodical Bibliography

The following articles have been selected to supplement the diverse views presented in this chapter.

Robert Bazell	"Tissue Issue," *The New Republic*, June 29, 1992.
Tim Beardsley	"Aborted Research," *Scientific American*, February 1990.
Sharon Begley et al.	"Cures from the Womb," *Newsweek*, February 22, 1993.
John Carey and Stephen Baker	"Brain Repair Is Possible," *Business Week*, November 18, 1991.
Council of Scientific Affairs and Council on Ethical and Judicial Affairs	"Medical Applications of Fetal Tissue Transplantation," *Journal of the American Medical Association*, January 26, 1990.
Glamour	"Medicine vs. Politics," March 1992.
Kim A. Lawton	"Curing or Killing?" *Christianity Today*, May 18, 1992.
Stanley M. Marks	"We Need a New Policy on Fetal Tissue Research," *American Medical News*, December 14, 1992. Available from 535 N. Dearborn St., Chicago, IL 60610.
Lance Morrow	"When One Body Can Save Another," *Time*, June 17, 1991.
Stephen G. Post	"Fetal Tissue Transplant: The Right to Question Progress," *America*, January 12, 1991.
Janice G. Raymond	"Taking Issue with Fetal Tissue," *On the Issues*, Spring 1993. Available from Choices Women's Medical Center, 97-77 Queens Blvd., Forest Hills, NY 11374.
Andrew Simons	"Brave New Harvest," *Christianity Today*, November 1990.
Carson Strong	"Fetal Tissue Transplantation: Can It Be Morally Insulated from Abortion?" *Journal of Medical Ethics*, June 1991.
Dick Thompson	"When Abortions Save Lives," *Time*, April 6, 1992.
Robert J. White	"Fetal Brain Transplantation: Questionable Human Experiment," *America*, November 28, 1992.
Kenneth L. Woodward et al.	"A Search for Limits," *Newsweek*, February 22, 1993.

4 CHAPTER

Are Reproductive Technologies Ethical?

Biomedical Ethics

Chapter Preface

Today, some doctors claim, it is not necessary for any family that wants a child to go without one—or more. The development of such techniques as artificial insemination, in vitro fertilization, cryogenic preservation of sperm and ovum, embryo transfer, hormone boosting, and sperm augmentation have made it possible for people until recently considered infertile to become the biological parents of children. Those with even more severe problems, such as a woman born without ovaries, can be helped through such practices as surrogacy, in which one woman bears a child for another.

For childless couples, these techniques may seem to be miracles unimaginable only a decade or two ago. But many people do not think these practices are as wonderful as they seem. Some opponents of the new reproductive techniques have philosophical objections. They say people have no business interfering in the work of nature—or God. Other opponents point out that these techniques pose physical and psychological dangers for many women. Enduring several operations in the hope of becoming pregnant can deplete a woman's health. Finally, critics point to the relatively low success rate of those who undergo extreme procedures. For example, according to some studies, only one woman out of twenty who undergo in vitro fertilization actually becomes pregnant and bears a healthy child.

To many childless couples, the opportunity to be the one in twenty is worth every moment of agony. To others, it is a deceptive and dangerous technique that ought to be curtailed. The authors in this chapter present several views of the new reproductive technologies.

"The idea of the new technology is, you bypass everything. . . . It's fantastic."

Reproductive Technologies Offer Hope to the Childless

Judy Berlfein

Artificial insemination, in vitro fertilization, hormone boosting, and surrogate gestation are just a few of the techniques available today to increase the possibilities of reproduction for childless people. In the following viewpoint, Judy Berlfein, a medical and science writer, discusses what some couples go through to overcome infertility. Despite the complexities and often low success rates of reproductive technologies, she says, many people wishing to have biological children view them as a source of hope.

As you read, consider the following questions:

1. What statistics presented by the author offer some explanation for the booming interest in reproductive technology?
2. According to Berlfein, are the new reproductive technologies "magical" solutions to the problem of infertility? Explain.

Judy Berlfein, "Searching for Fertility," *Los Angeles Times*, October 6, 1991. Reprinted with permission.

Sarah Bromley [all patients' names have been changed] lies on the operating-room table, fading into a state deeper than sleep. Nurses place sheets across her body, leaving an opening over a small section of her lower abdomen. The surgeon, Dr. Joel Batzofin, uses a scalpel to cut a tiny hole in her navel. He inserts a long tube through the incision, pumps Bromley's abdomen full of air and then attaches a video camera eyepiece to the outer end of the tube. A nurse fiddles with a monitor beside Bromley, and, as the screen vividly reflects each move the surgeon makes, suddenly the "Fantastic Voyage" is no longer just Hollywood invention.

"Here is the uterus and the Fallopian tube," Batzofin dictates into a microphone as his surgical tools manipulate the slippery interior of the body. "Notice the scarring on the tube from the ectopic pregnancy," he says.

Another object appears on the screen—a catheter filled with fluid, a liquid containing three potential human lives. The catheter slides into the opening of the Fallopian tube, and Batzofin continues his dictation: "We are placing three embryos into the left Fallopian tube."

Bromley is undergoing zygote intra-Fallopian transfer, or ZIFT, one of several variations on the test-tube baby-making theme, in which a zygote, meaning a fertilized egg or embryo, is transferred from a petri dish to a Fallopian tube. If all goes well, nature takes over, carrying the embryo to the uterus.

It is Bromley's third attempt at ZIFT at Pasadena's Huntington Reproductive Center, where Batzofin serves as co-director. The first procedure resulted in an ectopic pregnancy, with the embryo settling in the inhospitable environment of the left Fallopian tube. The second was a success, but Bromley miscarried several weeks into the pregnancy.

Fourteen days after the third procedure—two weeks of waiting on pins and needles—Bromley is greeted with more bad news: None of the embryos took hold in the uterus.

Alternatives to Infertility

Bromley isn't alone in her quest or her heartache. One in six couples in the United States has trouble conceiving a child, according to RESOLVE, a national support group for infertile couples. And although the number of people struggling to have a baby has not increased, the congressional Office of Technology Assessment's 1988 report on infertility disclosed that the number of people seeking treatment nearly tripled between 1968 and 1984.

Twenty years ago, when a couple had trouble conceiving, they were left with essentially very few options: adopt, or remain childless or take a chance on the relatively new field of infertility medicine. Today, medical advances keep pace with the demand for help and provide couples with more than a handful of choices. With these alternatives, however, an intimate process once confined to one's own home has moved to the laboratory and mushroomed in complexity, leaving parents-to-be both hopeful and confused.

Reproduction Landmarks

Landmarks in reproductive technology:

1799 Pregnancy reported from artificial insemination.

1890s Artificial insemination by donor.

1953 First reported pregnancy after insemination with frozen sperm.

1976 First commercial surrogate motherhood arrangement reported in the United States (surrogate is artificially inseminated and paid to carry child for an infertile couple).

1978 Baby born after *in vitro* fertilization (IVF) in the United Kingdom.

1980 Baby born after IVF in Australia.

1981 Baby born after IVF in the United States.

1983 Embryo transfer after uterine lavage (female donor is artificially inseminated but embryo is flushed out of her uterus and transferred to waiting recipient).

1984 Baby born in Australia from embryo that was frozen and thawed.

1985 Baby born after gamete intrafallopian transfer (egg and sperm are mixed and injected into Fallopian tube).

First gestational surrogacy arrangement reported in the United States (woman who gives birth has no genetic tie to child).

First reported pregnancy after fertilization of frozen egg.

1986 Baby born in the United States from embryo that was frozen and thawed.

1989 Baby born to oldest reported patient—49-year-old menopausal woman—to undergo one of the advanced reproductive technologies (embryo from husband's sperm and a donor egg is transferred to woman).

Source: "Infertility: Medical and Social Choices," Office of Technology Assessment.

Moreover, though statistics have improved since Louise Brown, the first test-tube baby, was conceived in 1978, success rates in the infertility business have been open to debate. For

155

example, while the Office of Technology Assessment estimates that as many as half of the couples seeking treatment came away without a baby, the American Fertility Society considers that figure overly pessimistic. The confusion results in part from the varying approaches to treatment by patients and doctors alike. Some couples may undergo only an initial workup at limited expense, while others are willing to exhaust all avenues, spending a small fortune in the process. At the same time, each physician will scale the ladder of potential therapies at a different pace and diagnose different conditions.

It's a course many people take haphazardly, not always grasping the ramifications.

Bogus Infertility Specialists

The average obstetrician-gynecologist has been trained to deliver babies and treat gynecological illnesses. Specialists in infertility undergo a two-year post-residency fellowship in reproductive endocrinology and infertility. As treatment becomes more popular and profitable, however, those without additional training are claiming infertility expertise.

Says Dr. Richard Marrs, director of the Institute for Reproductive Research at the Hospital of the Good Samaritan: "You can go into any city, into any medical building, and the majority of OB-GYNs today list themselves as obstetricians specializing in OB-GYN and infertility."

Marrs, who is a reproductive endocrinologist, believes that many physicians are overextending themselves at their patients' expense. "There are a lot of people who do obstetrics-gynecology and infertility who really should know their limitations— when to pass a patient on to a more sophisticated level of treatment," he says. "I wouldn't have the foggiest notion of what to do with a patient who is in premature labor at 34 weeks. I don't keep up with that literature; I don't do obstetrics."

Obstetrician-gynecologists, however, treat women, and women represent only half of the infertility equation, a point that the medical Establishment has overlooked for years. When a couple experienced difficulty in conceiving, the physician focused on the woman and, for the most part, neglected the man.

"I certainly think that there's a general realization that the male has been sort of having a free ride," says Dr. Howard Jones, founder of the Jones Institute for Reproductive Medicine at Eastern Virginia Medical School. In the last few years, however, more urologists are receiving training in andrology, the study of male reproduction, allowing specialists to place equal emphasis on both partners. In facilities such as Huntington Reproductive Center, Batzofin and his partner, Dr. Paulo Serafini, both reproductive endocrinologists, work side by side

156

with andrologist Dr. William Blank.

Once a couple decides on a team of doctors, they must consider all the potential treatments. How much can they afford to spend? How many different drugs are they willing to subject themselves to? How far will they go before calling it quits?

Initially, both the man and woman will be examined for clues explaining their inability to conceive. The routine procedures include a sperm test for the man, hormone evaluations for the woman and tests to assess the compatibility of the sperm with the vaginal environment. If problems are detected, physicians often recommend surgery, medication, insemination (the injection of sperm directly into the uterus) or a combination of the three.

If none of these help, couples can try assisted reproductive technologies. The most common are in vitro fertilization (IVF), first performed in 1978; the more recent gamete intra-Fallopian transfer (GIFT), and ZIFT, the operation Sarah Bromley underwent. In IVF, the egg is fertilized in a petri dish but placed directly in the uterus, not a Fallopian tube. The GIFT technique transfers a mixture of the egg and sperm to a Fallopian tube.

While these new methods have allowed many couples to achieve parenthood, their success rates still remain low. According to the scientific journal *Fertility and Sterility*, in 1988 only 12.1% of the IVF procedures in the United States produced a baby; the figures for GIFT and ZIFT, respectively, were 21.2% and 20%.

The Miracles of Test-Tube Baby-Making

Still, many physicians have more faith in the miracles of test-tube baby-making than in their understanding of the roots of infertility. Dr. Sherman Silber, author of "How to Get Pregnant With the New Technology" and director of in vitro fertilization, GIFT and microsurgery at St. Luke's Hospital in St. Louis, says, "I think that in 90% of cases, we really can't be too confident at all that a diagnosis we come up with is anything other than a normal variant that we would see in fertile couples."

The prime example Silber cites is endometriosis, which he says many doctors use as a catch-all explanation for infertility. The term is a derivation from endometrium, the lining of the uterine wall. In a diseased state, endometrial cells proliferate outside the uterus, growing on the Fallopian tubes, ovaries or lining of the abdominal wall.

In severe cases, such growth can damage the tubes or infiltrate the ovaries, physically interfering with pregnancy. Many cases, however, are mild, and in these situations, there is controversy over treatment. Silber frowns on those routinely prescribing medication and surgery. "When you look at all the data," he says, "there's been a tremendous over-diagnosis of endometriosis. Half the women who are diagnosed don't even have it."

Kathy Smithers has been coming to Huntington Reproductive Center for four months. She and her husband, Ken, have been on the baby chase for three years now. Today, she is propped up on the table and covered by a sheet, ready to undergo an ultrasound procedure. Dr. Paulo Serafini inserts a probe into her vagina and moves it slowly from side to side. He's on an egg search, hoping that the doses of Pergonal Kathy has been taking have stimulated her body to produce more than the single egg nature normally provides. He points to a few darker shades of gray on the screen, counting the developing follicles that house the eggs. One ovary has been prolific; the other side reveals nothing.

Badly Wanted Children

Despite all the problems engendered by the new reproductive methods and their uses, they have the potential of helping many infertile couples to have children. It is hard to object to this. These children are badly wanted and greatly prized in a world where this is too often not the case.

Marcia Angell, *New England Journal of Medicine*, October 25, 1990.

Kathy will return tomorrow, possibly with Ken but, more important, with a small cupful of his semen. The sperm will be spun in a centrifuge, separated from the seminal fluid and then injected into her uterus. The intrauterine insemination—also known as IUI—of washed sperm, often combined with fertility drugs such as Pergonal or clomiphene citrate to stimulate ovulation, is one of many treatments that has become commonplace in the infertility regimen.

Many physicians swear by it, and any woman spending more than a few months with a fertility specialist will probably undergo her fair share of inseminations. Logically, it would seem to increase the chances of conceiving. Rather than forcing the sperm to travel the precarious pathway through the acidic environment of the vagina, the sperm are placed directly in the uterus, significantly closer to their destination in the Fallopian tube.

Inseminations often serve as a bridge between assisted and non-assisted reproductive technologies. If nothing else is working, many specialists believe that a trial of inseminations ranging from $200 to $1,200 per shot may be more sensible than a GIFT or IVF procedure, costing $4,000 to $10,000.

But a small minority of specialists protest the blanket use of insemination. "We think it's appropriate," Marrs says, when the sperm are slow or weak or handicapped in some manner. This extra boost might result in fertilization. "It's probably of no benefit in any other situation in fertility," he adds. Nonetheless, women receive inseminations routinely regardless of the exact diagnosis.

Silber agrees with Marrs: "I haven't seen any studies that prove that [the procedure] creates a higher pregnancy rate than just timed intercourse with clomiphene citrate or Pergonal. And yet it's very common."

Batzofin doesn't dispute these allegations. "Perhaps there are not enough adequate, well-controlled studies to prove that they work in given situations," he says. "Yet we do them a lot because they do work. Sometimes it's unethical to withhold treatment, in the name of objectivity, just because the definitive scientific study has not been done."

High-Tech Options

Batzofin ushers David and Julie Ferguson into his office. David has undergone a varicocele ligation, an operation to improve the quality and quantity of his sperm. Unfortunately, however, after a series of inseminations, Julie still hasn't become pregnant.

Frustrated and at a loss, the couple ask Batzofin to outline the high-tech options. They have been conservative long enough, David seems to concede. Julie leans forward in her chair in a "let's not beat around the bush" gesture. She wants the details, the specifics and the costs. They are both 37 years old and sense time tugging at their heels.

Some proponents of high-tech fertility methods argue that patients spend too much time and money finding out that the low-tech treatments won't work for them. If couples attempted GIFT, ZIFT or IVF earlier, doctors say, they might succeed sooner and come out ahead financially.

"You can come up with a lot of different diagnoses and treat them, spending literally a fortune on conventional methods of treatment," Silber says. "Whereas the fact is, if you look at age, there is just an age-related decrease in the ability of a woman to get pregnant." The prime years of reproduction for women, most physicians agree, fall during the early 20s. After that, fertility simply declines.

Silber believes that most infertility specialists are driven to find a diagnosis, to offer an explanation to the patient. But in reality, he says, doctors have very few answers to offer. When it comes down to it, it's simply hard to get pregnant. "The idea of the new technology is, you bypass everything," Silber says. "It's fantastic."

Other physicians might disagree with Silber's advocacy of high-tech treatments. They say these approaches, which can run between $4,000 and $10,000, should be reserved only for last-resort patients, those without any remaining options.

"I have a certain concern," Dr. Howard Jones says, "that high-tech treatment is being used in a large number of patients who have unexplained infertility. That suggests to me that therapy is being applied before a precise diagnosis is made."

In Julie and David's case, however, Batzofin doesn't push. He simply tries to make the options clear. He's pleased with Huntington Reproductive Center's success rate in assisted reproductive technologies and presents the statistics. Since Julie's Fallopian tubes are intact, he suggests ZIFT, the procedure with the most encouraging statistics. With the center's averages almost double the national figures, there seems to be cause for guarded optimism. The national pregnancy rate with ZIFT is 20%; the center's rate is 41%.

Knowing these numbers should make the couple's decision easier. But behind every figure is another question. While Huntington Reproductive Center's figures include all women under age 40, statistics elsewhere may be based only on "good candidates," those with limited obstacles to pregnancy. So how do these numbers translate to Julie and David's particular situation?

"It's very difficult to find populations that are completely equal in order for you to compare," says Dr. Ricardo Asch, director of the Center for Reproductive Health at UC Irvine. "It's all a little bit relative. We give our clinical judgment according to our experience. There is not a mathematical formula that you put in the computer—the patient age, sperm count, years of infertility, tests performed—and then the computer spits out a treatment. It's more your feeling, what your clinical experience tells you to recommend."

As David and Julie weigh their decision, there is still hope—but a weariness, too. Julie considers the next hurdle, the 50-50 chance that she will come away this year with a baby or another disappointment. Her no-nonsense, straight-to-the-facts approach melts away as the tears well up.

She has sought answers and received qualified maybes. Certainty remains an elusive concept. As with any pregnancy, old-fashioned or high-tech, creating a baby will ultimately require the same ingredients: a bit of knowledge and a great deal of luck.

"If we refuse to take a hard look at how we are using the new technologies, we may allow women's reproductive lives to be deformed in frightening ways."

Reproductive Technologies Offer False Hope and Serious Risks

Barbara Katz Rothman

Although reproductive technologies such as in vitro fertilization seem to offer hope to the childless, author Barbara Katz Rothman asserts in the following viewpoint that the hope they offer is minimal and the health risks involved are high. Rothman, a professor of sociology at City University of New York and the author of *Recreating Motherhood*, contends that those involved in the fertility business are more interested in making a profit than in either the physical or psychological welfare of the hopeful patients, most of them women.

As you read, consider the following questions:

1. Rothman says, "Reprotech . . . rarely delivers." What are some of the statistics she uses to back up this statement?
2. What are some of the dangers of reproductive technologies noted by the author?
3. What "brave new world" of the future does Rothman fear if reproductive technologies are not checked?

Barbara Katz Rothman, "The Frightening Future of Baby-Making," *Glamour*, June 1992. Reprinted with permission.

The wall behind the receptionist's desk is covered with baby photos: a four-by-six-foot testimony to success. You have to look carefully to notice that the little redhead at the bottom is also in the "first Christmas" photo in the corner; the infant twins on the left are also grinning toothily on the right. Actually, there aren't all that many babies. But for someone who has been trying and trying and *trying* to conceive, the photos overwhelm.

This is the entrance to a typical high-tech infertility treatment center. The baby photos are an effective sales pitch for a rapidly proliferating array of reproductive technologies. In vitro fertilization (IVF), which brought Louise Brown into the world, is now only one ingredient in an alphabet soup of baby-making. Besides IVF—letting sperm and egg join in a petri dish before continuing growth in utero—there's now GIFT (gamete intrafallopian transfer), ZIFT (zygote intrafallopian transfer), TET (tubal embryo transfer), PZD (partial zona dissection), MESA (microsurgical epididymal sperm aspiration) and more, all used or combined in the attempt to create pregnancies. The new term technologists use to cover the whole package of infertility techniques is assisted reproductive technologies, or ARTs. Some refer to it more casually as reprotech.

If you read only the literature offered by the clinics—or the newspaper and magazine articles that parrot their claims— reprotech is about helping women have the babies they want.

In truth, reprotech is deeply problematic. It subjects women to techniques that have not been carefully evaluated. It is rarely successful—at best, one out of ten women who go through these procedures ends up with a healthy baby. Reprotech reinforces some of our most backward attitudes about women, and its social implications are chilling.

This revolution is occurring in the near absence of legal controls. What regulation does exist is chiefly focused on protecting embryos and fetuses from the negative effects of experimentation, not women or the children and families that will be. Yet the new technologies will soon become a routine part of baby-making for *all* women—not just infertile ones—ultimately limiting rather than expanding our reproductive choices.

Shattered Hopes

Reprotech promises babies; it rarely delivers. Clinics routinely claim success rates of around 25 percent, but most often *success* is defined as a pregnancy—not a healthy baby.

Recently, because of pressure from clients, some centers have begun to advertise their "take-home-baby rate. " Even there, the numbers are misleading. The percentage given is "per transfer"—that is, the number of babies resulting from a certain number of transfers from a petri dish to a woman's womb. But many infertile women never get as far as producing an embryo for transfer; they drop out of an IVF program because they do not ovulate, even with the fertility drugs they're given, or they ovulate, but the eggs never become fertilized. *These women are not counted in the total when success is measured per transfer.*

Furthermore, per-transfer statistics tell how many babies are created—not how many mothers. Four babies among 20 women sounds like a 20 percent success rate, unless you know that the four were two sets of twins. Or one set of quadruplets.

Of course, any woman may be one of the lucky ones—the one in ten—who gets a baby. Will the child be healthy? According to Robert Lee Hotz, author of *Designs on Life*, figures from IVF clinics around the world show that IVF has produced five times the normal rate of babies with spina bifida and six times the normal rate of those with transposition, a serious heart defect. An IVF baby is three times more likely to die in the first three months of life. (The results of technologies other than IVF are too new even to have been tabulated.) Keep in mind that, given the high cost of IVF, these are babies of relatively affluent parents who have good access to pre- and postnatal care.

Despite their photos of smiling babies, then, IVF centers aren't producing a lot of happy mothers. The norm isn't a success story but a giddy cycle of hope and disappointment or even despair. Researchers report that many women experience months or years of exhaustion, depression and debilitating side effects because of the procedures.

The Health Risks

The cost of the new technologies to would-be parents is not just financial or psychological. Reprotech employs invasive treatments involving powerful drugs and surgery, and deaths do occur. Gena Corea, author of *The Mother Machine*, has uncovered over a dozen reprotech-related deaths (in at least one case, the woman's ovaries burst due to overstimulation by fertility drugs) and many more instances of life-threatening reactions to the procedures.

Although the new technologies are now primarily aimed at infertile women, one of the latest uses is in the treatment of *male* infertility. A favored new technique is microinjection—injecting a single sperm into an egg in a petri dish in cases where a man's sperm is sluggish or he cannot ejaculate (in the latter instance, the sperm is surgically extracted from the testes). But while using the fertile sperm of *another* man—donor insemination—offers a couple a more than 80 percent chance of becoming parents and does not increase the risks to the woman's health, microinjection has the same 10 percent success rate as other IVF procedures. And like other IVF procedures, it increases the risk of ectopic pregnancy, which can *cause* female infertility. Thus a woman who has undergone IVF treatment because her partner is infertile may find that when it fails, as it generally does, she has developed tubal adhesions that could eliminate donor insemination as an option.

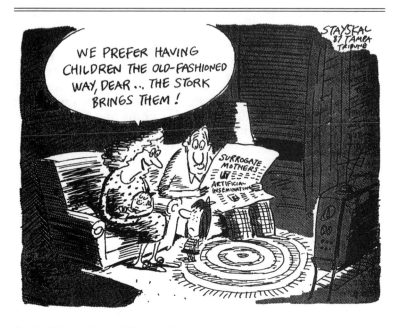

Reprinted by permission: Tribune Media Services.

But it is what the doctors call the "theoretical but unproven" risks that cause the most worry. Marsden G. Wagner, M.D., of the World Health Organization's Copenhagen office has already expressed concern that fertility drugs may lead to cancer in women—after all, the drugs stimulate rapid cell growth, the hallmark of that disease. Ann Pappert, a journalist who has been interviewing reproductive technologists around the world, says that even they are worried. One renowned specialist told her bluntly: "We expect a cancer epidemic." And now that researchers have learned that clomiphene citrate (Clomid), one of the drugs used to stimulate ovulation, can linger in the woman's body for weeks, exposing the fetus to powerful hormones, the possibility of a DES-like tragedy in the next generation looms.

Comparing reprotech with another recent popular technology—breast implantation—reveals some interesting parallels. Both technologies exploit women's deep need for something that promises to make them "real" women: large breasts, a baby. With both, doctors have been only too glad to profit from this need while shutting their eyes to foreseeable health risks and telling themselves they're contributing to female well-being.

Even less research has been done on the risks of reprotech than on those of breast implants. As with breast implants, no central records are kept to monitor potential problems. A study funded by the National Institutes of Health is only now beginning to follow up on 5,000 women who have undergone reprotech since 1988. The study has not met its goals for recruitment of subjects, and if it does not get renewed funding from NIH next year, it may be abandoned.

It's not even accurate to say that women treated with the new technologies are participating in an experiment. In an experiment there are controls. And there are reports of results.

A Technology Out of Control

Reprotech is an industry driven by the lure of scientific "progress" and the promise of profit. It is not primarily concerned with the long-term welfare of women.

The United States, with its free-market ideology, has traditionally been reluctant to interfere with the development and sale of scientific services. In addition, health care has been considered the business of citizens, not government: The U.S., almost alone among industrialized nations, lacks a national health program. Our federal government has no power to directly regulate medical services. *There is no federal board authorized to review embryo experiments.*

And as abortion has become a politically explosive issue, the federal government has grown more wary of getting involved in any legislation having to do with fetuses. Regulation has fallen to the states, which license health care personnel and facilities. Most of the state laws now on the books are designed to protect fetuses; they stipulate that once an embryo is created through reprotech procedures, it may not be discarded.

These laws have resulted in some absurdities. Reprotechnicians try to fertilize several eggs at one time, since many will not take. Before freezing was available, any extra embryos that were created had to be implanted. Although doctors generally *wished* to implant some extra embryos, to increase the likelihood of a successful conception, large multiple pregnancies threatened the woman's health and put the embryos in the classic "lifeboat" position: If all remained, all might die. Hence pregnancy reduction: the selective aborting of some of the embryos. It was illegal to discard the embryos when they were in a petri dish, *but not once they were inside a woman's body.*

Embryo freezing was supposed to solve this problem. Today,

couples can try for a successful pregnancy again and again with less stress, danger and expense than before because new rounds of hormonal stimulation to produce eggs are no longer necessary. The flip side: There are now thousands of embryos stocked in freezers worldwide. What of the ethical dilemmas when their "parents" divorce or die?

Because no regulatory body is wrestling with the snowballing medical and ethical questions created by reprotech, the market provides the only limits to its expansion. By the time most people have thought through the possible fallout, we'll be living with it.

Not for Women's Health

New reproductive technologies such as in vitro fertilization, embryo transfer, gamete-intrafallopian transfer, and so on, do not contribute nor are they meant to contribute to women's health. For that matter, neither do contraception, sterilization, nor abortion—which have increased the incidence of infertility—contribute to women's health. The question that the Royal Commission faces is this: What kinds of health risks is Canada willing to subject its women to in order to allow new reproductive technologies to help them have the children they want? This is a much more difficult question than whether or not a particular technology is in the best interest of a woman's health. If the Commission dealt with the latter problem, its task would be easy. But an immeasurably more difficult task is forced upon it when women express their willingness to expose themselves to serious health risks in order to have a chance of conceiving a child by means of a new reproductive technology.

Donald DeMarco, *Fidelity*, July/August 1991.

The dearth of regulation doesn't mean that the new technologies have developed in a random fashion. The techniques that have been invented and the way they've been used have been shaped by an age-old, male-centered way of looking at reproduction.

Surrogacy contracts already declare that some pregnant women are not mothers but simply rented space. Motherhood has been separated into two parts, the genetic and the gestational, and it's the genetic component—the component that's equivalent to what the father contributes—that is considered the more important. Some states already issue birth certificates that list the egg donor as the legal mother and omit the name of the woman who bore the child, as if she did no mothering at all.

Many women desperately want a child that is biologically

theirs, or at least their partner's. They are willing to undergo the stress, expense and possible health risks of reprotech for the slim possibility that they will end up with a child with a blood tie. Such a heartfelt need cannot be dismissed. Is it possible, though, that the need may not be "natural" but social? Western society has always put genetics above nurturance, not least so that men would be able to control the transmission of property from one generation of males to the next. But we should consider that our obsession with the biological connection may backfire on future generations.

For if we refuse to take a hard look at how we are using the new technologies, we may allow women's reproductive lives to be deformed in frightening ways. The technologies don't have to work any better than they have been to become standard practice. Just remember breast implants. General anesthesia was widely used for childbirth even though it endangered both mothers and babies; doctors recommended bottle-feeding even though it increased infant mortality; DES was used to prevent miscarriage even though it didn't work (and eventually was shown to be the cause of grievous birth defects).

Frightening Scenarios

It's not hard, therefore, to imagine the turn things will take in the near future. Already, fertilized eggs, like sperm, can be frozen and stored indefinitely. And reprotechnologists are working on freezing *unfertilized eggs*. Commercial frozen-egg banks are likely to follow; the following reproductive counseling session might be nothing out of the ordinary:

June 15, 1997

"Yes, Joan, you and Tom are both carriers for cystic fibrosis. You can, of course, just take your one-in-four chance of having a child with this disease. You'll need to check if your insurance company still covers voluntarily created birth defects, though. You could adopt. [Here the counselor's voice drops.] A few years ago, I'd have suggested getting pregnant, aborting if prenatal diagnosis showed the fetus was affected. It was very hard on the parents, but it was a choice. Now, well, I'm not supposed to discuss abortion with you, so if you want to pursue that option, you'll have to try another state. [The counselor's voice resumes its normal level.] Another possibility, Joan, is to have you inseminated by another man. Or you could have Tom's child, using donor eggs. After all, you'll still be carrying Tom's baby, and that's what counts, isn't it? Let's just fill out this form for the Humpty Dumpty Frozen-Egg Bank. "

Once the technology of egg-freezing for "medical reasons" is firmly in place, it is bound to proliferate. All of our reproductive technologies have followed this path. It's been true of bottle-

167

feeding and also of amniocentesis, which has led to greater health risks for fetuses (infection, spontaneous abortion). It's been true of fetal monitoring and ultrasound, which have led to a rise in unnecessary cesareans.

"Choice" Can Become Compulsion

How else might egg-freezing come to be used? Consider that in the Gulf War, the military was rumored to have toyed with the idea of using drugs to halt menstruation in women soldiers. Five percent or more of the female crew on at least one Navy vessel came back from that war pregnant—so those in charge might well be more aggressive with a fertility-control plan *next* time. . . .

"Choices" have an alarming way of becoming compulsions. Birth control, for example, was an option women fought hard to obtain. Now it's hard to imagine a woman choosing *not* to regulate fertility. In today's economy, who can afford families of eight children? While birth control is quantity control, the new push is toward quality control—screening to prevent the birth of babies with disabilities and diseases. Sometimes this is a way of sparing our potential children great pain and suffering. But it is also a way for parents and society to avoid the economic costs of raising children with disabilities. Genetic screening is already experienced as a given by many women, who feel it will be their fault—and that they will get little social support—if they deliver a "defective" baby. Once the technology of embryo biopsy is widely available, *all* women may face what I envision for Helen:

June 15, 2007

"Of course, Helen, you can go ahead and get pregnant with Frank any old way. But is that sensible, mature? Let's run you through three cycles over the next few months, extracting eggs, fertilizing them with Frank's sperm and freezing them. We'll grow the embryos for a bit, test them and use only the very best. This is the most important decision of your life. You wouldn't have accepted any husband by chance—why should you accept any embryo?"

I've limited myself here to fairly conservative scenarios. Others—ethicists, theologians, lawyers, even some reprotechnologists—have predicted more radical ones for the next 20 years:

• Parents-to-be choosing their babies from catalogs—prefabbed embryos, cloned and ready for implantation.

• Reproductive brothels, where the embryos of wealthy couples from all over the world are gestated in the bellies of poor American women. European and Asian couples already come here to hire surrogates.

• Removing ovaries from aborted female fetuses so that eggs may be harvested before the contamination of living can touch them. The result: armies of laboratory creations growing in the wombs of animals or in machines, humans without human parents.

Even the tamest of these scenarios would produce drastic changes in the meaning of parenthood and family. One of the most likely, ironically, would be a new devaluation of pregnancy and motherhood. If we continue to offer only minimal financial and emotional support to mothers and families, if we continue to value competition and achievement over nurturance, will a lawyer or surgeon of the next generation want or be able to "waste time" on pregnancy? Wouldn't it be easier simply to farm out gestation (not to mention mothering) to low-paid "reproductive workers"?

Mother and Child, or Manufacturer and Product?

We are already coming to think of parents, especially mothers, not as sources of nurturance but of contamination. As the fetus is increasingly seen as a product and a woman as its housing site, we focus on all that can be "toxic" about that site—does the mother smoke or drink? Eat junk food? Soon we're on the road to the artificial womb as the ultimate solution to the problem of imperfect parents. There is also the experience of children to consider in this brave new world. The more we see children as products we can design to our liking, the more they will be constricted by our expectations and perceive themselves as objects meant to fulfill *our* particular needs, rather than as intrinsically valuable human beings.

The reproductive technologists, caught up as they are in the wonders of the quest to make babies out of raw materials, seem to have forgotten these dangers, lost sight of the meaning of parenthood, made children almost irrelevant. At a recent conference on the new technologies, one doctor from IVF Australia presented data on the application of reprotech to women well past menopause. I sat openmouthed, no longer a sociologist but my eight-year-old self whose father had unexpectedly died. What do these scientists think it might mean to have parents facing the serious problems of aging while their children are cutting their molars? What about the inevitable orphanhood of so many of these children? Do scientists see no connection between the cells they implant and the real, living child that is created?

A Braver New World

The new reproductive technologies are not inherently bad. They *can* give women more control and more choice. The goal is to change how we are using them.

"Technological reproduction . . . promotes medical profiteering, professional ambition, and clinical adventurism over the bodies of women. "

Reproductive Technologies Harm Women

Janice G. Raymond

Janice G. Raymond is a professor of women's studies and medical ethics at the University of Massachusetts, Amherst. She is a founding member of the National Coalition Against Surrogacy and the author of many books and articles on reproductive technologies and other women's issues. In the following viewpoint, Raymond asserts that far from being motivated by sympathy for the infertile, those who promote reproductive technologies do so at the expense of women. These technologies, she states, endanger women's lives and demean women by giving primacy to the rights of men and of the fetus.

As you read, consider the following questions:

1. Raymond claims that infertility did not spur the development of reproductive technologies; rather, the technologies led to the promotion of infertility as a problem. What does she mean? What do you think of this argument?
2. The author asserts that the new reproductive technologies place the woman in the position of least importance in the vital quadrangle of woman-man-fetus-technology. Do you agree with her argument? Explain.

Janice G. Raymond, "International Traffic in Reproduction," *Ms.*, June 1991. Reprinted with permission.

They claim it all started with infertility—thousands of desperate couples clamoring for a technology to have babies. But it really started with the technology itself. On the first day, reproductive experts created the technology of in vitro fertilization; on the second day, the script of infertility. As scientist Erwin Chargaff confirmed, "the demand was less overwhelming than the desire of the scientists to test their new techniques. The experimental babies produced were more of a by-product."

Like religious fundamentalism, medical fundamentalism has a determining set of principles. The first principle of new reproductive dogma is that infertility is a disease and technological reproduction is the cure. But technological reproduction does not "cure" infertility: it only provides children to a small percentage of couples—mostly white, middle-class, married, and heterosexual.

Reproductive Fundamentalism

In vitro fertilization (IVF) was the showcase technology in whose glow all the other newer reproductive technologies basked: offshoots such as GIFT (gamete intrafallopian transfer) and ZIFT (zygote intrafallopian transfer); superovulation and TUDOR (transvaginal ultrasound-directed oocyte recovery); fetal reduction; embryo transfer; surrogacy; embryo and egg freezing; fetal tissue transplants; fetal surgery; postmortem cesarean sections—to name a few.

A second principle of new reproductive fundamentalism is that any technique that might produce pregnancy can be tried on so-called desperate, baby-craving women. No matter that most reproductive technology is experimental and destructive to women's bodies, that 90 to 95 percent of the women who undergo in vitro fertilization never take home babies, that in other areas of medical treatment such a failed technology would only be used in life-threatening circumstances.

The ideology of infertility is based on a double standard. If infertility is genuinely the concern of reproductive medicine, why is it not doing something to stop the greatest cause of infertility in the world—mass sterilization of women in developing countries? Third World countries have long been a dumping ground for chemicals and drugs discredited in the West—DDT and DES, for example. The Pill was initially tried on women in Puerto Rico. The Dalkon Shield, taken off the market in most First World countries, remains implanted in many Third World women.

Women in Brazil and Jamaica were among the first tested in the Norplant trials. Norplant is the contraceptive implant that remains embedded under a woman's skin for about five years; it generated such problems in Brazilian women that feminists, in

171

cooperation with a government study committee, succeeded in canceling the trials—for a time. Yet when Norplant was approved by the FDA [Food and Drug Administration] for use in the United States, the Brazilian data was not evident.

Infertility in Perspective

Is there a real problem of infertility in the West? Infertility caused by environmental pollution and sexually transmitted diseases (STD), as well as medically induced infertility such as pelvic inflammatory disease (PID) caused by IUDs [intrauterine device], is on the rise. IVF experts report an epidemic in the West, with one out of six or seven couples being infertile. Yet both the U.S. National Center for Health Statistics (NCHS) and the U.S. Office of Technology Assessment (OTA) contend the more accurate figure is one in 12. Their studies show no increase in the number of infertile couples between 1965 and 1982.

What has changed is the *definition* of infertility. There is no scientific consensus, but the currently accepted definition is inability to conceive after one year of intercourse without contraception. Recently, the number of years has dwindled from five to two to one, thereby confusing the inability to conceive with difficulty in conceiving quickly.

The media portrayal of infertility and the infertile is deceptively simple and homogeneous. Those undergoing IVF are portrayed as forever infertile, whereas a large percentage of "infertile" women have had children in a present or a previous relationship. Many undergo IVF because their husbands are infertile. It has been estimated that 25 percent of women on IVF programs are there because of male partners' problems. Many gynecologists never order analysis of the husbands' sperm. And frequently, men are reluctant to be tested.

The number of office visits to physicians for infertility services rose from 600,000 in 1968 to 1.6 million in 1984. The only infertility epidemic is of fertility specialists; between 1965 and 1988, membership in the American Fertility Society jumped from 2,400 to 10,300. Scientists and doctors with ordinary backgrounds become reproductive virtuosos. Alan Trounson, a well-known Australian IVF expert, began work as a sheep embryologist. He then applied this knowledge to humans; now, Trounson has taken the IVF techniques he learned on women to breed goats.

In Vitro Fertilization

In vitro fertilization is the basis for all the rest of the technologies. Once the egg and sperm are placed in a petri dish, doctors can freeze embryos, transfer them from one woman to another, determine their sex, and use them for experimentation and genetic manipulation. Initially a "fringe" technology, IVF is now regarded as the most conservative of new reproductive procedures.

Over 200 U.S. institutions performing IVF treatment have been established. In the absence of federal funds for research in this area, the tab has been picked up by patients, pharmaceutical companies, universities and hospitals, and private organizations often relying on venture capitalism. A large number of these centers are for-profit "fertility institutes" that perform other reproductive services such as surrogacy and sex predetermination as well. Although rates vary, a conservative cost estimate is about $5,000 per IVF cycle. Many women return for two, five, and sometimes ten cycles.

Damaging Effect on Families

The desire of a married couple to give visible expression to their love by conceiving and bearing a child is among the most basic and noble of human aspirations. The frustration and sense of emptiness which accompany the recognition that the desire may never be realized can lead a couple to an uncritical acceptance and use of the developing reproductive technologies. Whether "successful" or not, use of these techniques can have far-reaching and damaging effects on the individual marriage partners, on their relationship and on their present and future life together. The presence and support of sensitive and compassionate family and friends can help the infertile couple appreciate the threats posed by these technologies. More importantly, they can help the couple to explore ways to address their suffering in ways which are life-giving and life-affirming.

Jean deBlois, *The Catholic World*, September/October 1992.

The U.S., however, is not the reproductive technology capital of the world. France has more IVF centers per capita than any other country; Australia has had the highest success rates, along with major government support. In Victoria, Australia, the 1985 budget allocated only Australian $25,000 for STD research and prevention, yet it financed $1 million of IVF expenditures. Australia has exported its IVF technology to the U.S. in a venture known as IVF Australia, which has set up many for-profit fertility centers in this country and elsewhere. But doctors in the U.S. are eager to join the entrepreneurial fray; for example, doctors who own Northern Nevada Center, an IVF clinic, believe that eventually IVF could be a $6 billion annual business.

Rarely has a technology with such dismal success rates been so quickly accepted. As Gena Corea and Susan Ince documented in 1985, half of the clinics reporting success never had a live birth. Some centers claimed success by using the number of implantations that never resulted in births or by the number of chemical pregnancies—the elevation of hormone level that may but often doesn't indicate an ongoing pregnancy.

In the U.S., there is still no accurate assessment of live-baby rates. The 1989 Wyden congressional subcommittee reported a 9 percent "take-home baby" success rate for IVF, but it noted that many clinics report success but do not mention live births. England's take-home baby rate is 8.6 percent; Australia's is 8.8 percent—but only 4.8 for healthy babies.

The number of healthy children born is another hidden statistic. A 1987 Australian government report noted an increase in premature births and low-birth-weight babies associated with IVF (26.9 percent for 1985), and revealed that the mortality rate of children in the first 28 days after birth was 47.5 deaths for every 1,000 births—four times higher than for non-IVF births. The report also documented that congenital abnormalities among IVF babies is greater than expected.

In fact, IVF's *lack* of success has been the justification for developing new technical variations. The problems of multiple fetuses due to superovulation and multiple implants, chronicled in a 1988 British report, are used to justify fetal reduction—also known as "selective termination of pregnancy." Doctors inject a saline solution into the uterus to abort some of the fetuses, which may cause bleeding, premature labor, and the loss of all fetuses or damage to any remaining.

When the technology may harm fetuses and children, people take note—but not when the harm occurs to women. Much of technological reproduction is a form of medical violence toward women: hyperstimulation of the ovaries and possible cysts frequently result from superovulation—as does immense pain and trauma. The medical literature treats these problems as mere technical imperfections—"collateral damage" as it's called in war. Gena Corea has documented the deaths of at least ten women in connection with IVF procedures. . . .

Sexual Politics and Reproductive Technology

The connection between sexual and reproductive politics is no mere metaphor. Jacques Testart, lab-parent of the first French IVF baby, Amandine, writes of his "incestuous" feelings: "I invested myself in a role that was not . . . paternal. I felt I was the lover, not the father. . . . I would like to discover her once she's a person . . . I see myself as a lover and not as a father."

In 1869, Josephine Butler condemned enforced medical examination of prostitutes mandated by the Contagious Diseases Acts then enacted in England; she called the exam instrumental rape by the steel penis. In the 1980s, an Austrian female student-

174

observer described the vaginal harvesting of eggs from a woman in full view of a medical school class: "At each follicle puncture he [the doctor] retracted the needle and then drove it in hard. The woman asked him to stop, because she was in great pain. But Dr. M. would have none of that . . . and so [more] follicles were punctured against her will . . . again each puncture unmistakably resembled a penetration."

More and more, the "old" sexual roles within which women have been confined converge with the "new" reproductive roles women are offered. The act of men buying women for sex bears a striking resemblance to men buying women's reproductive services in surrogacy. Surrogate brokers are reproductive pimps. The men who hire women as surrogates have their own specific reproductive proclivities they will pay extra for, such as insemination with only Y-bearing sperm or amniocentesis for "quality control" of the product. . . .

Threat to Women's Rights

Technological reproduction is sometimes included in the pro-choice platform—as if these technologies promote women's reproductive rights. Feminists who oppose technological reproduction have been accused of undermining reproductive rights, especially abortion. Yet the exact opposite is true: feminist *support* of technological reproduction threatens women's right to abortion.

The new reproductive technology spotlights fetuses and would-be fathers' rights. "Rights" of fetuses and would-be fathers are augmented, while this technology challenges the one right that women have historically retained some vestige of—mother-right. The extent to which the rights of women are diminished when the fetus is part of the woman's body should make us seriously question the extent to which they will be further diminished as technology increasingly removes the fetus from the female body.

We witness an assault on women's rights in surrogate custody and frozen embryo disputes in which the rights of "ejaculatory fathers" are presented as their rights to gender equality (or, as the fathers' rights movement phrases it, "Equal rights are not for women only").

The right to choose is fast becoming the right to consume. Women are supposed to become consumers for new technologies and drugs—for more and more dangerous ones in the case of technological reproduction. Of course, all women and all feminists do not agree on the dangers. Some contend that women can use these developments for their own purposes and that feminist critics portray women as helpless victims incapable of using these options in their self-interest. And besides, some say, the new technologies are inevitable.

Fortunately, there have been many women's groups who do recognize these abuses. . . .

In the U.S., the Institute on Women and Technology, founded to bring a feminist perspective to public policy on technologies that affect women, joined with ex-surrogates at federal and state legislative hearings to testify against bills that would permit or permissively regulate surrogate contracts. The institute advocates legislation making such contracts legally void and unenforceable. Another institute project documents the incidence of IVF-related deaths of women worldwide; called the Zenaide Project, it is named for a Brazilian woman who died as a result of IVF procedures.

Those who advocate technological reproduction, claiming sympathy for the infertile, offer a shortsighted solution that fails to extend the same sympathy to the thousands of Third World women who are rendered infertile by mass sterilization and contraceptives. It neutralizes the violation of women inherent in these technologies, while appearing to be sensitive to women. And it promotes medical profiteering, professional ambition, and clinical adventurism over the bodies of women. Such sympathy serves mainly to strengthen a society in which women, reproduction, and motherhood are continuously created in the image of man and medicine.

"Not all women are against IVF, and not all women feel abused by IVF."

Women Want Reproductive Technologies

Lene Koch

Lene Koch, a research fellow at the department of social pharmacy of the Royal Danish School of Pharmacy, Copenhagen, teaches women's history and writes extensively on women's issues. In the following viewpoint, Koch summarizes a study she did of women seeking in vitro fertilization. Koch, an opponent of IVF, discovered that many women, even those knowing the potential harms of IVF, looked to this technology as a solution to their infertility. Koch asserts that it is important to recognize and respect these women's motivations.

As you read, consider the following questions:

1. Besides the desire for a baby, for what reasons do women turn to IVF, according to the author?
2. What alternatives does Koch seem to think are better than IVF?
3. How does the author say feminist critics of reproductive technologies should address women's desires for such procedures?

From Lene Koch, "IVF—An Irrational Choice?" *Issues in Reproductive and Genetic Engineering*, vol. 3, no. 3, (1990). Reprinted by permission of Pergamon Press Ltd., Oxford, England.

One of the most difficult problems that have confronted feminist critics of in vitro fertilization (IVF) and the other new reproductive technologies is the great enthusiasm for IVF among involuntary childless women. In spite of concerned feminists' dedicated public exposure of the low efficiency and high risks of IVF, involuntary childless women—the target group of IVF—do not seem to listen. Instead they gather in IVF centres where they form long waiting lists, organize in groups lobbying local and national politicians to finance more IVF clinics, and stand up at public meetings to denounce feminist criticism of IVF. How should feminist IVF critics interpret these women's active conscious support and enthusiasm for IVF? The dilemma caused by this enthusiasm is an urgent one, since critical feminists claim to present a view representative of the interests of women while a politically crucial group of women publicly represent the opposite view. "Women want it" has often been the argument of IVF supporters. Now it has become the argument of the involuntary childless women themselves. . . .

There is no doubt that IVF is a powerful transformer of women's reproductive consciousness and an irresistible technology that few women can refuse. It is also beyond dispute that feminist studies such as Renate Klein's [1984 study] have documented the gross neglect, malpractice, and false information that many IVF practitioners are responsible for, and which only feminist criticism seems capable of exposing. But even if we disregard the fact that, for example, Klein's selection of women is limited to those who have finished a programme *without* a child, and for that reason we may be expected to be more negative towards IVF than a representative sample of women, these women's lack of proper information about IVF is interpreted as the main reason for their feeling of being abused—"broken by patriarchy," as Klein puts it. But, as Eva Fleischer has noted, it would be doubling the tragedy to regard these women as victims only, or solely coerced, since there would be no way out of the situation: "How can women decide against IVF, if they are totally dominated by patriarchy, even in their innermost feelings?" Though neglect, abuse, and misinformation are widespread, they do not constitute the solution to the feminist dilemma.

A New Medical Technology

Methodology. My own interviews were undertaken as part of a larger study to evaluate IVF as a new medical technology. Fourteen women participated in the study. Women were contacted through the Danish State Hospital in cooperation with the IVF clinic at this hospital. Forty-five women on the waiting list who were to begin treatment in January 1987 received a letter of invitation to participate in the survey. Fifteen women responded positively. One left the waiting list before the survey was undertaken. Each woman was interviewed three times; once before, once during, and once after the final IVF attempt. . . .

Another Look at "Facts"

Information. The interviews kept bringing up remarks and utterances that left me only partly satisfied with earlier explanations. A number of the women I interviewed were quite ignorant of both chances of success and risks of IVF. But some knew almost everything there was to know. As one cycle followed another, more and more women obtained a more realistic view of their chances. But still they continued treatment with great zeal and energy. In a number of cases, the women felt deprived of correct and realistic information, but regardless of the amount or quality of information received, somehow *information did not matter*; it did not seem to have influenced these women's decision either to start IVF in the first place, or to continue after one or more failed attempts. In spite of the fact that most women had been presented with information about their chance of success, only a few were able to reproduce this information. The statistical information about clinic results that the women had been given by the hospital were often transformed in the minds of the women to suit their subjective expectations. These expectations varied a lot from woman to woman, and basically mirrored the individual woman's self-confidence. The reason each woman gave for believing in success did not base itself on "objective facts," but rather on her own subjective "magical" belief that she was particularly suited for IVF, or that she was bound to be lucky.

Knowledge about the objective statistical chance seemed to be less important than the mere fact that there is a chance. No matter how negligible this factual chance is, it must be tried. This particular "logic" forms an important part of the explanation why information is of less importance.

One woman puts it this way: "Factual information was unimportant to me. Even if they had told me I had a chance of 0.5%, I would have believed in success, naturally." Another example of the "irrational" approach to the facts of IVF relates to the risks of the treatment. Side effects of the hormonal doses that are used to superovulate were rarely complained of. All women were affected by inconvenient or painful side effects. But at the same time several women expressed content with these side effects. "Then I know that the hormones have had an effect" was a typical remark.

Pain is an important part of IVF, and IVF-women's willingness to stand the pain is one of the things that surprise feminist critics. But we should remember that most women who try IVF have been through a number of infertility treatments that are both painful and require medical intervention. All women in my survey had had operations and before that most had several cases of PID [pelvic inflammation disease], often caused by abortions or use of an IUD [intrauterine device]. These women have already put a great strain on their bodies. The pain of IVF is only a slight additional pain in the larger scheme to resolve infertility.

Several women, who had been told about the increased risks of twins and triplets, still preferred to have a multiple pregnancy in spite of the risks. This attitude was related to the fact that IVF is only offered to childless couples. If IVF succeeds once, there is no chance of another child through publicly financed IVF. It may seem odd that women are not frightened by the possibility of twins or triplets, even if they know the risks, but examples as this show that the logic of both critical feminists and conscientious doctors is not always compatible with the logic of infertile women in IVF programmes.

Anger and Discontent

Feelings. The anger and discontent of women who failed IVF is a prominent theme in Renate Klein's survey. And certainly, anger would be a natural response to one or more failed attempts of IVF. In my survey some women were angry because the treatment did not result in a child or because they were treated without human sympathy, but just as many were not possessed by negative feelings towards doctors and clinic. One had an abortion, had a subsequent depression, and was in strong need of therapeutic help, and expressed great dissatisfaction that she did not get any help from the hospital. But the large majority were content. Their points of criticism were often stated in constructive ways as good ideas for the clinic to think about. Furthermore, the majority were happy they had had the opportunity to try IVF, and would not have been without it. To them IVF was not a violation of their human dignity. They rather considered IVF an offer every woman should have access to—a human right in fact. And in spite of the pain and anguish that most women reported, they would recommend IVF to a friend and would themselves start all over again. Naturally, most of them failed to leave the clinic with a child, but somehow this failure was not always considered synonymous with the feeling of a wasted effort. "I have reaped what there is to reap" was the comment of one woman who left the programme without a child after three IVF cycles. The controversial question: Do women want IVF? was thus answered in the affirmative by the majority of the women in my survey.

I set out defining the feminist dilemma: Why do women choose IVF in spite of low success and high risk? But I soon realized that my way of putting the question was different from the way the women would have done. They did not try IVF "in spite of," they did it "because of." They continually answered my questions: "Why did you choose IVF?" and later: "Why do you continue IVF?" with this simple statement: "Because I want a child." To want a child and try to have it is an exercise of the reproductive freedom that the feminist movement has argued for since its very beginning. The decision to have a child at age 30 may be seen as a natural succession to the decision to contracept at 18, to have an abortion at 20; in other words, to avail oneself of the medicotechnical services of the health system—first to avoid having a child, later to have one.

A Woman's Choice

If women want to try technological solutions to their reproductive problems, we may be unhappy about the risks they could be taking with their own health; if women want to avoid bearing children suffering from a particular disease, we may have fears about the implications for society. But we feel that women, and women alone, should be the ones to make the choice. That still leaves room for us to hold views as to how we hope those choices will go, to enter debate on the issues raised and to struggle to make the conditions under which reproductive choices are made less constraining.

Lynda Birke, Susan Himmelweit, and Gail Vines, *Tomorrow's Child: Reproductive Technologies in the 90s*, 1990.

The wish for a child has often been commented on by those of us who are critical of the new reproductive technologies. This wish, we argue, is socially constructed, and should not be considered a biological need. We state that there is a contradiction between society's priority of medical solutions to infertility and the socially constructed wish for a child. The research that has been undertaken to demonstrate this contradiction in health policy decisions is of great importance sociologically and politically, but it leaves out an important problem; unless we accept a view of women who seek IVF as mere victims of social norms and influences, the nature of the wish for a child for the individual women must be considered an *authentic wish*. The wish for a child does not become less strong and authentic because it is socially constructed. The fact that infertile women want children, want to have a so-called normal family, is part of the explanation of why they do not hear the feminist critics. What they instantly perceive, however, is that most of the feminist critics do

181

not find children "necessary" to live a good and satisfying life. Several studies rightly present the alternative of "child-free" lives as important to develop and strengthen. But the woman who has not resolved her infertility or come to terms with it psychologically does not hear this. To present infertile women to an analysis of infertility as a social construct will most likely lead to total rejection of such feminist ideas. Furthermore, infertile women do not consider prevention of infertility a relevant alternative to IVF. This is an option for future generations—not applicable to their situation. This then is the plain explanation why women try IVF in spite of all the feminist warnings: *The wish for a child is an authentic wish.*

Why Don't Women Behave as Rational Beings?

A number of questions still persist: Even if women authentically want a child, why don't they behave *rationally?* We have seen that women say yes to IVF in spite of its low success rate, in spite of the side effects of the hormones, in spite of the risk of multiple births. But why do they say yes to IVF when they KNOW all this? . . .

Both anthropologists and philosophers have participated in the debate on the nature of rationality. One view is that the common use of the concepts of rationality/irrationality covers more than the mere question of logical consistency. One important issue is related to the question of criteria of rationality cutting across cultural differences. Are so-called "primitive tribes" less rational than we are, because they believe in magic and witchcraft? Or are we more rational because we live in a culture based on modern technology and science that is able to send a man to the moon? . . .

The cognitive-instrumental rationality is characteristic of the work of technology and science. The most important criterion of validity is efficiency—the successful result. This relates to the instrumental power that this type of knowledge wields. In contrast to this stands the subjective-expressive rationality of the individual. Its criteria of validity are relative and may simply be subjective honesty. The specific rationality, for instance, of women seeking IVF relates to the structure of their subjective worldview and is disconnected from concepts like intelligence and logical thought. Differences in rationality may be caused by different worldviews. If we apply this line of thought to our present problem, it seems possible to consider the worldview of IVF women as belonging to a culture structured by its own rationality, its own logic and own purposes.

If we accept the thesis that women who try IVF make their decisions and experiences on the basis of their own specific worldview structured by their specific rationality, we still need to understand the principles of this rationality.

This understanding must be based on the reproductive situation of the infertile woman. All women in my survey had been through years of treatment including medical examinations, hormonal treatments, operations. To most, IVF was just another possibility in the series of medical treatments of infertility. With the arrival of IVF on the reproductive market, most women felt they had to try, even though they had almost given up hope. To resolve their reproductive future, they had to pass IVF—as a "rite de passage" as Sarah Franklin has put it. In this context, the physical and emotional pain of IVF may be considered a ritual, an ordeal that has to be experienced.

Social Stigmatization of Infertility

Most women experience infertility as a loss of control, an experience that is often reinforced by social stigmatization of infertility. The decision to try IVF—may be considered an attempt to liberate oneself from the powerlessness of infertility—if only to realize that a child of her own is no longer an issue. I am not talking of a decision undertaken after rational calculations of costs and benefits, but a decision that invests the woman with the feeling of having done what was necessary, and thus having an impact on her life. Even though IVF is an experience that makes many women feel helpless and out of control, this is being balanced by the empowering act of having chosen, having decided to take advantage of existing opportunities. This decision is often made in anticipation of regret at a later point in life, out of fear to regret that one did not try everything when the opportunity was available. As the third and last attempt of IVF draws to a close, all women in my survey express a feeling of relief. They all look forward to the moment when they will leave the IVF-programme. "Liberation," "peace of mind," and "great relief" are the expressions that the women use to characterise the situation when IVF will be ended definitively. This relief is expressed by all, regardless of the result of IVF, including those who do not accept that IVF is over once their opportunities in the public health care system are exhausted. [The Danish public health care system offers three completed cycles of IVF. After these have been finished, the woman must either accept her infertility or buy her way into a private IVF clinic.] Most women accept their infertility once they leave the public health care system. Two were unable to stop however, and travelled to England to continue treatment at their own private cost. Even these women considered it an advantage if they had been able to stop.

As mentioned above, the rationality of feminist critics (and science and technology, for that matter) has been exclusively oriented towards the explicit objective of IVF. Since the objective is to have a child, it seems irrational to choose IVF, since IVF only rarely leads to the desired objective. But the woman's decision to go along with IVF as well as her experience of the treatment itself, may be understood as an attempt to reach a secondary objective as a necessary substitute, that is, protection against social stigmatization and a means to obtain social recognition as an involuntary childless woman. IVF may be considered a way to prove to *others* that you are infertile—and is the precondition to a final resolution of infertility.

We may understand this as a consequence of the impact of IVF on the general perception of infertility. As each new reproductive technology enters the market, the definition of infertility changes. Infertility can only be defined as the condition that no reproductive technology can resolve. Thus, IVF virtually becomes an imperative, even for those women who might otherwise have been ready to accept their infertility. . . .

Naturally, women's desire to try IVF is primarily motivated by the chance to take home a baby. But, as I believe the presentation of my survey has shown, this is not the only motivation. "IVF—the chance to have a baby" constitutes a game—a ticket to a lottery—and only she who has played this game and lost, can establish a socially accepted identity as involuntary childless. Thus, the infertile woman not only judges IVF by its dubious capacities to let her have a child, but also as a new element in the procedure by which the woman establishes her future identity. . . .

Attitudes Toward IVF

My discussion has intended to show that when infertile women do not seem to hear the well-argued and well-founded warnings against IVF, then one explanation might be that these women have good reasons to go along with IVF, reasons that *we* don't seem able to hear. These women are different from us, live in other worlds, have other norms, and rationalize their thoughts and acts in ways different from us. The belief that some views are "right" and others are "wrong" will not bring us closer to a better world for women.

Let us, by using these women's self-defined "rationality" as our starting point, develop alternative ways of dealing with the wish for a child, and not be afraid to display cultural worlds and ways of thinking and acting that are different from our own. Not all women are against IVF, and not all women feel abused by IVF—no matter how hard we try to interpret their experience. Women act in many different ways, ways that rarely coalesce and often contradict each other.

"Surrogacy creates ardently wanted life. Morally speaking, this is the decisive factor."

Surrogate Mothers Contribute a Valuable Service to Society

Peter H. Schuck

In 1987, the well-publicized case of Baby M drew the public's attention to the practice of surrogate mothering, in which one woman bears a child for another. In the case of Baby M, the surrogate mother decided that she could not, after all, give up the child she had contracted to bear for another couple. Lengthy and costly court proceedings were left to determine the fate of the child. While several other prominent surrogacy cases have been in the news, hundreds of surrogacy cases have gone unchallenged and have created happy families. In the following viewpoint, Peter H. Schuck, Simeon E. Baldwin professor of law at Yale Law School in New Haven, Connecticut, argues that surrogacy can be a beneficial practice for society.

As you read, consider the following questions:

1. What are the advantages the author says surrogacy has over adoption?
2. What is the major reason Schuck believes surrogacy is an ethically sound practice?
3. How does the author think society can minimize the risks associated with surrogacy?

Peter H. Schuck, "The Social Utility of Surrogacy." Reprinted (sans footnotes) with permission from the *Harvard Journal of Law & Public Policy* 13 (Winter 1990): 132-38. Copyright 1990, Harvard Society for Law and Public Policy, Inc.

Surrogacy lends itself to a battle of abstractions. It inevitably invites combatants to invoke concepts like nature, natural rights, inalienability, personhood, and slavery. The peculiar political divisions among and between self-proclaimed liberals, conservatives, feminists, and libertarians on the surrogacy issue suggest to me that these concepts do little analytical work. Instead, they serve as empty vessels into which almost anything can be poured. I will therefore try to avoid this difficulty by evaluating surrogacy in terms of what we know about human sentiments, the social consequences of surrogacy, and techniques for controlling its genuine risks.

My position is that surrogacy can be a morally acceptable response to the deepest, most poignant human needs. If permitted and properly regulated by law, the social benefits that flow from surrogacy are likely to be immense. Although some risks are involved, they can be minimized by using standard regulatory techniques and specifically enforcing some but not all provisions of surrogacy agreements.

Although I will be addressing the topic of surrogate motherhood, I should note that the sale of sperm, which is quite routine under existing legal arrangements, raises many, but not all, of the same questions as surrogate motherhood. Yet interestingly enough, we have very few moral qualms about the donation or commercial sale of sperm. We must bear this in mind when assessing the moral arguments against surrogacy.

Background Assumptions

Before assessing those moral arguments, the social consequences of surrogacy, and the techniques for controlling its risks, let me state some of my background assumptions. I begin with the incontrovertible proposition that infertility is a personal calamity of enormous dimensions. According to the best data on the subject, infertility is increasing. In the United States, for example, one out of even six couples of childbearing age is infertile, and a very large percentage of those infertile couples desperately wants to have children.

A second morally relevant fact is that adoption today is considerably less available than it was in the past—even the recent past. Some reasons for this are the increase in abortions, the increased availability and use of contraception, and the reduced stigma of bearing children out of wedlock. Between 1971 and 1982, the number of legal adoptions each year dropped from 82,000 to 50,000. During the same years, a sharp decline occurred in the proportion of agency adoptions relative to so-called independent adoptions. Even as we speak, new impediments to adoption are increasing. In short, adoption is a diminishing solution to the problem of infertility.

With these facts in mind, I turn now to consider the moral status of surrogacy. First, we cannot doubt that surrogacy is baby selling; the assertion to the contrary made by the trial judge in the *Baby M* case was simply disingenuous. Surrogacy, however, is baby selling with a difference. It is different because the strictures against baby selling that arise in the adoption context do not necessarily condemn baby selling in the surrogacy context. Quite to the contrary, surrogacy advances some of the same values that the ban against baby selling in the adoption context is designed to promote. As with sperm or egg donation or sale, however, we seem to have very few moral qualms about adoption.

Helping Someone Else: Surrogates Speak Out

"If I was doing this for the money, I would have given up a long time ago," said Dawna, a 32-year-old woman who insisted that her last name not be used. "I just like being pregnant and I like the idea of helping someone else have something so special." She had three daughters and did not want to raise any more children when she became a surrogate for a New York City couple two years ago. . . .

"This is the most wonderful thing you can do for someone else," said Ali Bellamy, who has a 3-year-old daughter, a 19-month-old son and will travel to New York during her next ovulation cycle to try to become pregnant for the Alexandrus, [an infertile couple]. She says she feels deeply for the couple, who have suffered three miscarriages, an ectopic pregnancy, an unsuccessful in-vitro fertilization and rejection by adoption agencies because they are considered too old.

Surrogate mothers, quoted by Lisa Belkin, *The New York Times*, July 28, 1992.

Yet surrogacy has several advantages over adoption from a moral point of view. First, with surrogacy the father and the adopting mother have the advantage of considerably more information about the natural mother, the surrogate, than is typically available in the conventional adoption case. Second, a surrogate mother—unlike an adopting parent or a mother who is placing a child up for adoption—knows from the outset that even as the fetus proceeds to gestation, she has no legitimate expectations of a continuing relationship with the child. Obviously, that is not in itself an answer to the phenomenon of maternal bonding. It suggests, however, that there is a psychological overlay to the relationship between a surrogate and the growing fetus that is decidedly different. According to some empirical evidence, this difference seems to account for the fact that a surrogate will not feel the loss as keenly as a natural mother often feels when placing her child up for adoption. Third, and perhaps most important, surrogacy, unlike adoption, is an arrangement that creates new life. It is not simply the reallocation of rights to existing children. It is a phenomenon that promises the creation of new, desperately wanted life.

Opponents often make natural law objections against permitting surrogacy. One form of this objection is that the surrogate is using her body to produce and nurture a child for a stranger, a use of her body that opponents consider to be profoundly alienating. In assessing that claim, note that a similar use of the body is being made by one who sells or donates sperm or eggs, both of which practices are increasingly common. I recognize that there are differences between sperm donors and egg donors on the one hand and surrogates on the other. The question, however, is whether those differences rise to a moral dimension. I think that they do not.

A Commercial Arrangement

A second kind of natural law claim against surrogacy emphasizes the fact that the surrogate is carrying the child for a fee; it is a commercial arrangement. Again, recall that eggs and sperm are sold and that state law sanctions those sales. We do not seem to have any moral objections to such sales, although they raise legal and administrative problems that must be addressed through regulatory means. That the service being provided by the surrogate is precious does not necessarily argue against allowing that service to be exchanged for a fee. Many things in life that are precious are produced for a fee, including health care, child care, and many other services.

A third type of natural law claim against surrogacy is that it is involuntary. Opponents of surrogacy point to the complex psychological relationship that occurs between the surrogate and the growing fetus, a relationship that creates feelings that no woman prior to this experience can anticipate. Thus, the argument goes, contractual consent can never really be informed consent. Empirical evidence, however, refutes these claims. Interestingly enough, most surrogates have already had their own children. They have been through the process of pregnancy. They know what feelings to expect. It may be true that after delivering the child, a surrogate may experience regret regarding her decision to enter into the agreement, but the possibility of regret is ubiquitous in life and accompanies many of the major decisions that we make. Further, it is possible to minimize the risk of regret by making improved information about the experiences of former surrogates available to women intending to become surrogates themselves. Many surrogates apparently conclude that having undergone the experience, they rather liked it and would do it again. They feel that they are performing a priceless, albeit compensated, service for people who desperately desire their own children. Some surrogates, of course, feel differently.

Surrogacy Creates Life

Surrogacy creates ardently wanted life. Morally speaking, this is the decisive factor in evaluating surrogacy. The benefit of children being born to parents who cherish them; the benefit of creating life that would not otherwise exist; and the benefit of allowing women who wish to become surrogates to reap both economic and altruistic rewards for bestowing one of life's greatest gifts—these considerations argue very strongly against the natural law attack on surrogacy. We should be very reluctant to censure on moral grounds a practice that generates these kinds of values.

It should also be relevant to our moral debate that there have been very, very few problems with surrogacy arrangements relative to the overall number that have been undertaken. We have read a great deal about the *Baby M* situation and a couple of others, but according to recent data, the number of instances in which problems have arisen is well under a dozen, notwithstanding that more than 600 surrogacy contracts had been entered into between 1988 and 1990.

I would now like to turn from what we know about surrogacy to what we can reasonably predict about its consequences. The appropriate context for evaluating these consequences is a legal regime that seeks to maximize the social benefits of surrogacy and minimize its social risks. The first question then becomes: How highly do infertile couples value the prospect of having a child? We have some evidence bearing on this question because we know that couples typically pay a minimum of $8,000 per child in the case of agency adoption and a good deal more in the case of so-called independent adoption. We also know that there are about 500,000 to 1 million infertile couples who are likely to seek adoption. The economic value of the benefits produced, in terms of couples' willingness to pay, must be many hundreds of millions of dollars. This estimate is a very conservative one because parents would be likely to pay a good deal more for a child with whom they have, as a result of surrogacy, a genetic relationship. In addition, surrogacy produces added value by reducing the amount of time needed to obtain a child.

Shifting the Burden of Proof

The massive benefits of surrogacy certainly do not resolve the moral question. They do not even resolve the utilitarian question. But they do suffice, I think, to shift the burden of proof to surrogacy opponents to justify withholding benefits of this kind and magnitude from people who are willing to pay for them and from the society that shares them. These benefits create a strong presumption that we should regulate surrogacy rather than ban it, especially if regulation can minimize its risks.

Regulating Surrogacy

Surrogacy's major risks are inadequate information and the possibility of people changing their minds as the child develops in the womb or after the child is delivered. These risks, however, can be minimized through straightforward regulatory methods. The state can, at relatively low cost, increase the amount and quality of information that individuals have concerning surrogacy, the obligations that will flow from surrogacy arrangements, and how those obligations will be enforced. It can require standardized contract provisions. It can reduce the considerable uncertainty that now surrounds the legal status of surrogacy contracts and the extent to which they will be enforced. The law must also protect the child from the risk of abandonment in the event that the people who entered into the surrogacy arrangement change their minds. If these measures are adopted, the residual risks of surrogacy are likely to be very low, especially when compared with the benefits.

A related, very important issue is the extent to which specific performance of the surrogacy contract provisions should be enforced by the law. The best way to approach this question is not on a categorical basis but provision by provision. There are certain contractual undertakings that we should not specifically enforce. For example, we should not specifically enforce the surrogate's obligation to surrender the child to the father. There are other contractual provisions, however, that I believe should be specifically enforced.

The crucial point to be made in conclusion is that surrogacy may potentially generate enormous individual and social values while posing minimal risks, which can be addressed through a limited regulatory apparatus. The principal obstacle to realizing such benefits is the legal uncertainty that presently envelops surrogacy. This uncertainty is something that the law can and should do something about.

"Commercial surrogacy is morally wrong and should not be permitted."

Society Should Not Condone Surrogate Mothering

Thomas Shannon

Among those who criticize the practice of surrogate mothering, the main arguments revolve around two issues: the commodification and consequent devaluation of women and babies and the commercialization—some say the prostitution—of childbearing. In the following viewpoint, Thomas Shannon, who teaches religion and social ethics at Worcester Polytechnic Institute in Massachusetts, summarizes the arguments against surrogacy.

As you read, consider the following questions:

1. Shannon says that surrogacy turns both surrogate and fetus into commodities on the same level as other commodities bought and sold on the free market. Explain why you agree or disagree with this argument.
2. What are the family-related problems the author believes surrogacy raises?
3. What is Shannon's attitude concerning the regulation of surrogacy?

Thomas Shannon, "Against Surrogate Motherhood." Reprinted with permission from the November 26, 1990, issue of *Christianity and Crisis*, © 1990 by Christianity and Crisis, Inc.

Surrogate motherhood, like in vitro fertilization (IVF), has re-structured the relationships among sexuality, reproduction, and the nuclear family. Commercial surrogacy in particular has had a profound impact on our mores and morals, our understanding of family and human commitment, and our perceptions of children. That much is clear.

What is not so apparent is any willingness to engage as a society in a sustained critical discussion of these social and personal effects. In the interests of furthering that discussion, therefore, I would like to examine the morality of surrogate motherhood.

As with IVF, my general orientation assumes three critical considerations: the continued disvaluing of women in our society; the more general cultural attempt to render value-free the human body, body parts, and the relationships between and among people (the legal contract is more and more becoming the model for human relations); and the pronatalist bias of our society. Unlike my judgment of IVF, however, my position on surrogate motherhood is, finally, unambivalent: The practice should be stopped.

Surrogate motherhood is fraught with many difficulties. Taken together, they add up to a negative moral judgment. Let's begin the list:

Commercial Surrogacy

Who is the mother? Typically in commercial surrogacy (and this is the model I assume throughout this article), a woman is contracted to be the genetic-carrying mother while the wife of the biological father assumes the role of the nurturing mother. What, then, are the claims of each of the parties? It is specious to argue that the biological claims of the genetic-carrying mother are invalidated by contract when the claim of biological paternity on the part of the genetic father is used to void any necessity of his legally adopting the child.

We can't have it both ways. Either biology counts for something and the genetic-carrying mother's claims count for something—as do the genetic father's—or biology counts for nothing, and contract is the only basis for any relationship.

Should the practice of surrogacy continue, the relation of the genetic-carrying mother to the child must be clearly defined, especially in the event of the separation or divorce of the genetic-nurturing father and nurturing mother. The issue is the well-being of the child, responsibility for her or his care, as well as the status of relations with half-siblings and half-grandparents.

Baby selling. When you walk into a store, select an item, hand money to the clerk, and receive the item and a receipt, you have purchased the item. You have not paid a clerk for her or his services, though, to be sure, part of the cost of the item goes to pay the salary. If someone takes the item from you, you can initiate a legal process. You paid for it, and it is yours.

This is exactly what happens in commercial surrogacy. A contract is established, money is exchanged, and the child changes families. The genetic-carrying mother is to make no more claims; the baby is no longer hers. The genetic-nurturing father now has the baby, and it is his. No one can take it from him. If someone tries, he can start a legal action.

In all other instances when something is transferred on the basis of a financial exchange, we call that buying and selling. I see no reason to exempt surrogacy. The payment is not a fee. The broker gets a fee and the genetic-carrying mother's health costs are covered. The sum of $10,000 (about $1.33 per hour, calculated for the duration of the pregnancy) is usually given to the mother when she produces a child that fits the contract.

That is buying and selling. And when such a procedure is applied to a human being, it is a total denigration of her or his personhood.

Commodification. Surrogacy contributes to the "commodification" of the person and the body. In applying to become a surrogate, a woman's personality can become a commodity. Because the candidate knows her personality can influence whether or not she becomes a surrogate, she can experience herself as an instrument, a means to enhance that decision. Thus her personality can become objectified and can contribute to her alienation.

Additionally what is of value in surrogacy is the body of the woman. More precisely, her uterus. What is critical is that she be fertile and healthy. Her status and worth are measured by her reproductive abilities.

Social stereotyping. The practice of surrogacy suggests that a woman's role and worth come primarily from her child-bearing capacity. A wife who cannot produce children is considered flawed, causing the husband to find a woman who can produce what he wants. The surrogate's value stems from her reproductive capacity, for which typically some proof is required.

While the role of mother is valuable and socially important— as is the role of father—that role does not constitute the essence of a woman or exhaust her potential. To continue to insist on such reductionism is to ensure the second-class status of women.

Surrogacy and Prostitution

Reproductive prostitution. Some writers have suggested that surrogacy is analogous to prostitution. In female prostitution, the woman sells or rents her body or body parts, the relation is impersonal, she is to do what she is told, her value or usefulness comes from her function, and she is to leave when she is told. If there is a pimp, he gets a share of the money. In surrogacy, the only morally relevant differences are that intercourse is technical and the woman is to become pregnant.

But while the similarity exists, the comparison is harsh. Consequently some have suggested that this analogy automatically puts the surrogate into a negative position because of the disapprobation of prostitution. Unfortunately, the surrogate does find herself in a comparable position. The point of the analogy is not to argue by name calling, but to ask whether there are valid points of comparison and, if so, to draw conclusions.

Other persons argue that prostitution is a woman's choice and must, therefore, be respected. The same would hold for surrogacy: It is her decision and even though it might be critiqued, it can't be faulted.

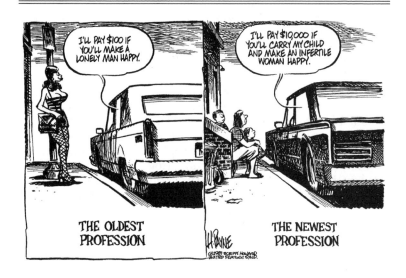

Henry Payne, reprinted by permission of UFS, Inc.

Such a position equates freedom of choice with the mere fact of choice and assumes no differences exist among objects of choice. Furthermore, the position assumes that the fact of being chosen makes the object of choice good or worthwhile. I would urge individuals who hold this position to think through the implications very carefully. Do we wish to equate autonomy with freedom to sell oneself?

Family implications. Other aspects of surrogacy, not always alluded to, relate to others intimately involved in the surrogacy process.

The children of a surrogate. While not all surrogates have children, having done so establishes the woman's fertility. If these children live with the surrogate, they will observe the pregnancy and its development. They will also observe that their half-sibling does not come home to live with them. Regardless of how this is explained, I fear such an event can have a detrimental effect on the children. We know that children have a variety of fears and anxieties about separation, about parentage, and about loss. Why fuel these fires?

The husband of a surrogate. Though not all surrogates are married, many are, and marriage is considered a desired sign of the woman's stability. But what is the motivation of a surrogate's husband or partner here? Can or should he just say "it's your decision; you deal with it"? Can or should either or both of them so neutralize their relations and their bodies that the pregnancy means nothing? Might there be a negative impact on their relationship from such efforts?

The wife of the genetic-nurturing father. While many women share in the desire to have a child and participate in the various reproductive technologies with their partner, the use of a surrogate might add a double sense of failure. Many women feel a sense of failure if they are unable to conceive and give birth to a child. If the husband then needs to go out and rent a woman to get a child, this might be a further blow to the wife's self-worth.

Another question involves the creation of a genetic asymmetry between the husband and wife with respect to the child. Should there be a death or divorce, could this genetic asymmetry be relevant in any arrangements made for the child? Such asymmetry might have more importance early in a pregnancy and in the initial years after birth. Later it might have diminished relevance because more traditional ways of resolving issues such as a custody dispute might be more easily applicable.

Women frequently assume the responsibility for soothing bruised male egos. A wife's cooperation with surrogacy may be yet another instance of such an unfortunate practice, yet another extra mile she may be willing to walk to let her husband satisfy his desire to have a child genetically related to him.

Regulatory Issues

As is the case with IVF, few regulations apply to surrogacy. Professional societies have made recommendations, which are fairly liberal. Only a few states have laws, and they vary. This situation needs immediate remedying.

Absolutely anyone may open a surrogacy clinic. With no experience in counseling, evaluating families, no medical expertise, I can start a clinic. And that scares me. Incentive exists to open a clinic. People are waiting to make use of such a service. Moreover, they are willing to pay not only the surrogate, but also the broker. Potential conflict of interest, therefore, needs to be resolved.

Additionally provision needs to be made for the interests of the child. What brings all the parties together is their desires: the desire to serve as a broker, to have a child, to be pregnant. And while all of these desires center on the child, what is paramount is the interests of all the other actors. Someone needs to ensure that the child's interests are protected.

But assume we have the perfect set of regulations and that everything that is appropriate is being done. We have counselors for all the parties involved, all kinds of screenings and evaluations; the mother does not change her mind. Am I, the critic, happy now? No, for efficiency or success is not an appropriate criteria for evaluating whether a practice is morally correct. Neither is the fact that we have regulations—even very good ones. Neither is the fact that no one ever changes her or his mind.

Surrogacy Is Problematic

Surrogates have to be screened for all kinds of physical and psychological strengths and weaknesses. They usually need post-birth counseling to help them respond to loss. All that suggests the practice of surrogacy is problematic. If we add to this the problems I have raised, the conclusion is inescapable: Commercial surrogacy is morally wrong and should not be permitted, regardless of the motivations and desires of the individuals involved.

Children are precious. They are our future. The development of reproductive technologies attests to people's strong desires to have children. But we need to be exceedingly careful that these desires do not lead us to adopt morally dubious practices.

Periodical Bibliography

The following articles have been selected to supplement the diverse views presented in this chapter.

Charlotte Allen — "When Motherhood Is for Sale," *The Wall Street Journal*, January 8, 1991.

Katrine Ames et al. — "And Donor Makes Three," *Newsweek*, September 30, 1991.

B. D. Colen — "Using Our Own Judgment," *Health*, January 1990.

Brian Doyle — "The Church Shouldn't Prohibit Test-Tube Babies," *U.S. Catholic*, June 1992.

Philip Elmer-Dewitt — "A Revolution in Making Babies," *Time*, November 5, 1990.

Diane Goldner — "Should I Donate My Eggs to Michael and Linda?" *Glamour*, January 1992.

Carolyn Helmke — "Surrogacy: Is It Just Another Labor Issue?" *The Guardian*, April 10, 1991.

Ellen Hopkins — "Tales from the Baby Factory," *The New York Times Magazine*, March 15, 1992.

Robert W. Lee — "Doing Everything Possible," *The New American*, September 10, 1990. Available from the Review of the News, Inc., 395 Concord Ave., Belmont, MA 02178.

Ruth Macklin — "Artificial Means of Reproduction and Our Understanding of the Family," *Hastings Center Report*, January/February 1991.

Dan Morris — "All We Wanted Was a Baby of Our Own," *U.S. Catholic*, February 1992.

Janice G. Raymond — "Reproductive Gifts and Gift Giving: The Altruistic Woman," *Hastings Center Report*, November/December 1990.

Should Animals Be Used in Research?

Biomedical Ethics

Chapter Preface

Well before the twentieth century, scientists discovered the efficacy of using animals in biomedical research. By using animals, scientists could discover the potential effects on human patients of various drugs and medical techniques without risking human life. A noble endeavor, many would say. But others disagree. They ask what right scientists have to exploit and harm animals to benefit humans. Those who disagree with the premise of animal experimentation point to laboratories where animals are crammed into tiny cages and given no opportunity to exercise or to socialize; where animals are implanted with cancer-causing agents, subjected to painful and lethal doses of chemicals, causing them to lose hair, skin, and sight; where they are purposely crippled or shot or maimed. Many of these atrocities, say animal protectionists, are committed in order to perform experiments that are redundant, unnecessary, or misleading—they will never be applicable to people.

However, many researchers disagree with the conclusions of those who would ban animal research. Diseases such as smallpox that decimated whole societies in earlier days have been all but wiped out because of animal-based research. Diabetics today can live normal lives because of the insulin developed through animal research. People who in past generations would have died early deaths from heart disease can today be saved because of animal research that allowed the development of cardiac pacemakers and artificial heart valves and the techniques used to implant them.

Some scientists hope that in the near future computer science will be so advanced that computer simulations will replace the use of animals in the research lab. That day has not yet arrived, however, and until it does, these scientists say, the continued use of animals is imperative to save human life.

The authors of the viewpoints in this chapter debate some of the issues centering on the use of animals in biomedical research.

"Had there been no experimentation on dogs, sheep and pigs, . . . I would have died."

Animal Research Saves Human Lives

Richard Pothier

Richard Pothier, a professional writer residing in Philadelphia, was the recipient of a heart transplant. That experience convinced him that human life is indeed more valuable than animal life. In the following viewpoint he points out that decades of animal research led to his successful transplantation surgery. He concludes that because the use of animal organs for transplantation offers additional hope to ill humans, animal research must continue.

As you read, consider the following questions:

1. The author contends he is an animal rights supporter, yet he is in favor of continued animal research. How does he say it is possible to be both?
2. Why, according to Pothier, is animal research necessary?

In a desperate—and successful—attempt to save the life of a dying man, woman, child or infant sometime in the next few months, surgeons will implant another heart or liver from a baboon or perhaps even a pig into a human body. Then, two things will happen. Doctors will decide whether the recipient will use the animal organ as a "bridge," until a human organ can be located for transplant, or if the patient will keep the animal organ as a permanent transplant. Second, animal-rights activists will picket the hospital where the medical miracle took place.

Twice in 1992, men dying of a strain of hepatitis that would most likely have destroyed a human organ received livers from baboons. Both times, the activists sprang into action.

Support for Animal Rights

I am an animal-rights supporter. I donate money to groups opposing some forms of medical experimentation on animals. I have argued for years, and will today, that animals are sometimes mistreated in such experiments.

But in my chest there beats a heart that used to belong to another person. Now it is mine, and it has already given me nearly four years of a complete and satisfying life after I fell victim to a deadly disease that destroyed my heart.

Had there been no experimentation on dogs, sheep and pigs, you would now be reading another essay by another person. I would have died in 1989. I almost *did* die at Temple University Hospital in Philadelphia until—just days before my shapeless, bloated heart would offer its last convulsive beat—a donor was found. I awakened from the operation with a strong, 27-year-old heart and a new life at the age of 49. Today, I am 53, healthy and happy. My ultimate life span is unknown. But so is everyone else's.

My doctors had to wait until almost the last moment before a suitable donor was found. But now, animal-to-human "xenografts" are nearing routine use as bridges to transplantations and promise a way to destroy the biggest killer in transplantation medicine—the deadly shortage of donor organs.

Americans refuse to donate enough organs to help the rest of us to stay alive. The number of heart transplants has peaked at about 2,200 a year. Thousands more of us could be saved from an untimely death. (About a third of recipients are under 44.) But the donor supply has plateaued. The reasons for this mystify transplantation experts. Twenty to 30 percent of those who need a heart transplant will die while they are waiting.

Biomedical engineers are working hard on mechanical replacements for hearts, but the human body does not take kindly to such machines. They present problems that may never be solved, and no mechanical solutions at all loom for bad livers, kidneys and lungs.

Anti-rejection drugs, however, can successfully allow animal organs to be used in humans. And there is hope that animal hearts, livers and perhaps even lungs could someday permanently replace diseased organs. In the future, genetically altered animals may be bred to provide matched organs for dying humans.

Animals Save Lives

Should animals be used in scientific studies? According to a report from the National Academy of Sciences Institute of Medicine, without animal tests "the world would be a very different place today."

The report notes that: "Many of us are here because we did not die as children, or our parents did not die, from diseases that have been controlled through knowledge gained from animal research."

And, despite the hue and cry from animal rights activists about the plight of animals, "even the animals that we keep as pets and raise for food would live shorter and less healthy lives, because many of the vaccines and treatments that have become staples of veterinary medicine would never have been developed."

John W. Merline, *Consumers' Research*, August 1991.

But this may never happen if animal-rights activists, with whom I agree on many things, convince society that it is wrong to sacrifice a pig or a baboon or a monkey to save a human. There are already numerous precedents for the use of animals to save lives. Insulin, which keeps diabetics alive, came from animal organs. Many Americans, including my mother, had their lives extended for years through the use of pig heart valves to replace their own faulty valves. I believe it would be a perversion of human sensibility to let infants, young people and men and women die prematurely, out of some bizarre belief that the animal has a greater right to life than the human.

New Heart

Both before and after I was diagnosed with cardiomyopathy, a lethal heart-muscle degeneration of unknown cause, I argued—and still do—that some medical experiments on animals were cruel and unnecessary. But before surgeons could implant a donor heart into my chest, they had to practice their skills on animals.

Do those opposing xenografts propose that surgeons practice

on people instead? Or that they don't practice at all? Before the surgeons sliced me open with a power saw and cut out my diseased heart, I had to know that I had good odds of awakening.

If my son should ever need the same procedure his father needed, and the disgraceful failure of many Americans to donate organs they no longer need continues to kill people, I hope *his* doctors will have available the option of saving his life with an animal's heart—either as a bridge to a human heart or as his own new heart. I want surgeons to learn their skills practicing on animals—not on my son.

If an activist needed a heart transplant, would he or she reject the use of an animal heart if that were the only organ available? Would he or she reject even a human heart, on the moral ground that thousands of animals had died to perfect this procedure?

Right now there are about 30,000 Americans waiting for a life-saving organ transplant. Every day more names are added to this list of desperate people. Among the newcomers are bound to be some of those who carry the protest signs or write the letters. It is one thing to come up with catchy phrases charging animal abuse; it may be quite another to die because your efforts at propaganda have been successful.

Animal organs can help fill the need. True, the medical problems of animal-to-human transplants have not yet been solved. But for at least 10 years, the problems of human-to-human transplants were not solved, either.

It may be tough for these well-meaning people to reverse themselves. But it will be tougher for them to carry their signs outside a hospital where a friend, or the child of a friend, is dying.

"Reasonable people should be able to agree on this: that alternatives to research that involves animal suffering must be vigorously sought."

Animal Research Is Unnecessary

Jean Bethke Elshtain

In the following viewpoint, Jean Bethke Elshtain cites several types of brutal animal research that she believes are unjustified. She asserts that most animal research does not lead to significant improvement in the human condition and that animals, having inherent value and dignity, should not be treated merely as objects. Elshtain, the Centennial Professor of Political Science at Vanderbilt University in Nashville, Tennessee, writes frequently on social issues and is a member of the Editorial Advisory Board of *The Progressive*, a monthly liberal magazine.

As you read, consider the following questions:

1. What facts does Elshtain offer in support of her contention that animal research is not justified?
2. What does the author say prevents the changes in research methods that might lessen dependence on animal subjects?

From Jean Bethke Elshtain, "Why Worry About the Animals?" *The Progressive*, March 1990. Reprinted by permission from The Progressive, 409 E. Main St., Madison, WI 53703.

These things are happening or have happened recently:
• The wings of seventy-four mallard ducks are snapped to see whether crippled birds can survive in the wild. (They can't.)
• Infant monkeys are deafened to study their social behavior or turned into amphetamine addicts to see what happens to their stress level.
• Monkeys are separated from their mothers, kept in isolation, addicted to drugs, and induced to commit "aggressive acts."
• Pigs are blowtorched and observed to see how they respond to third-degree burns. No pain-killers are used.
• Monkeys are immersed in water and vibrated to cause brain damage.
• For thirteen years baboons have their brains bashed at the University of Pennsylvania as research assistants laugh at signs of the animals' distress.
• Monkeys are dipped in boiling water; other animals are shot in the face with high-powered rifles.

The list of cruelties committed in the name of "science" or "research" could be expanded endlessly. "Fully 80 per cent of the experiments involving rhesus monkeys are either unnecessary, represent useless duplication of previous work, or could utilize nonanimal alternatives," says John E. McArdle, a biologist and specialist in primates at Illinois Wesleyan University. . . .

Even people who recoil from hunting and other abuses of animals often find it difficult to condemn such experiments as those cited at the beginning of this viewpoint which are, after all, conducted to serve "science" and, perhaps, to alleviate human pain and suffering. Sorting out this issue is no easy task if one is neither an absolute prohibitionist nor a relentless defender of the scientific establishment. When gross abuses come to light, they are often reported in ways that allow and encourage us to distance ourselves from emotional and ethical involvement. Thus the case of the baboons whose brains were bashed in at the University of Pennsylvania prompted the *New York Times* to editorialize, on July 31, 1985, that the animals "seemed" to be suffering. They *were* suffering, and thousands of animals suffer every day.

Alternatives Must Be Sought

Reasonable people should be able to agree on this: that alternatives to research that involves animal suffering must be vigorously sought; that there is no excuse for such conditions as dogs lying with open incisions, their entrails exposed, or monkeys with untreated protruding broken bones, exposed muscle tissue, and infected wounds, living in grossly unsanitary conditions amidst feces and rotting food; that quick euthanasia should be administered to a suffering animal after the conclusion of a

205

pain-inducing procedure; that pre- and post-surgical care must be provided for animals; that research should not be needlessly duplicated, thereby wasting animal lives, desensitizing generations of researchers, and flushing tax dollars down the drain.

What stands in the way of change? Old habits, bad science, unreflective cruelty, profit, and, in some cases, a genuine fear that animal-welfare groups want to stop all research dead in its tracks. "Scientists fear shackles on research," intones one report. But why are scientists so reluctant to promote such research alternatives as modeling, in-vitro techniques, and the use of lower organisms? Because they fear that the public may gain wider knowledge of what goes on behind the laboratory door. Surely those using animals should be able to explain themselves and to justify their expenditure of the lives, bodies, and minds of other creatures.

Animal Research Not Reliable

Lawrence Carter, director of the Health Care Consumer Network, says that "the AMA's [American Medical Association] attempt to identify animal rights activists as anti-science and against medical progress" is particularly galling. "I have cerebral palsy," says Carter. "To say that I'm opposed to medical progress is not only insulting, it's insane. What I question is the efficacy of animal-based research. The AMA won't tell you about drugs like Oraflex, which, although it was pronounced 'safe' after being tested on primates, caused liver damage and death when it was given to humans."

Phil Maggitti, *The Animals' Agenda*, June 1990.

There is, to be sure, no justification for the harassment and terror tactics used by some animal-welfare groups. But the scientist who is offended when an animal-welfare proponent asks, "How would you feel if someone treated your child the way you treat laboratory animals?" should ponder one of the great ironies in the continuing debate: Research on animals is justified on grounds that they are "so like us."

I *do* appreciate the ethical dilemma here. As a former victim of polio, I have thought long and hard for years about animal research and human welfare. This is where I come down, at least for now:

First, most human suffering in this world cannot be ameliorated in any way by animal experimentation. Laboratory infliction of suffering on animals will not keep people healthy in Asia, Africa, and Latin America. As philosopher Peter Singer has argued, we already know how to cure what ails people in desperate poverty; they need "adequate nutrition, sanitation, and health care. It has been estimated that 250,000 children die each week around the world, and that one quarter of these deaths are by dehydration due to diarrhea. A simple treatment, already known and needing no animal experimentation, could prevent the deaths of these children."

Second, it is not clear that a cure for terrible and thus far incurable diseases such as AIDS is best promoted with animal experimentation. Some American experts on AIDS admit that French scientists are making more rapid progress toward a vaccine because they are working directly with human volunteers, a course of action Larry Kramer, a gay activist, has urged upon American scientists. Americans have been trying since 1984 to infect chimpanzees with AIDS, but after the expenditure of millions of dollars, AIDS has not been induced in any nonhuman animal. Why continue down this obviously flawed route?

Third, we could surely agree that a new lipstick color, or an even more dazzling floor wax, should never be promoted for profit over the wounded bodies of animals. The vast majority of creatures tortured and killed each year suffer for *nonmedical* reasons. Once this abuse is eliminated, the really hard cases having to do with human medical advance and welfare can be debated, item by item.

Finally, what is at stake is the exhaustion of the eighteenth-century model of humanity's relationship to nature, which had, in the words of philosopher Mary Midgley, "built into it a bold, contemptuous rejection of the nonhuman world."

Confronted as we are with genetic engineering and a new eugenics, with the transformation of farms where animals ranged freely into giant factories where animals are processed and produced like objects, with callous behavior on a scale never before imagined under the rubric of "science," we can and must do better than to dismiss those who care as irrational and emotional animal-lovers who are thinking with their hearts (not surprisingly, their ranks are heavily filled with women), and who are out to put a stop to the forward march of rationalism and science.

We humans do not deserve peace of mind on this issue. Our sleep should be troubled and our days riddled with ethical difficulties as we come to realize the terrible toll one definition of "progress" has taken on our fellow creatures. . . .

I, for one, do not believe humans and animals have identical rights. But I do believe that creatures who can reason in their own ways, who can suffer, who are mortal beings like ourselves, have a value and dignity we must take into account. Animals are not simply a means to our ends.

207

"If we want to defeat the killer diseases that still confront us . . . the misguided fanatics of the animal-rights movement must be stopped."

Animal Rights Protesters Disrupt Valuable Research

John G. Hubbell

A "roving editor" for *Reader's Digest*, John G. Hubbell has written on a variety of topics. In the following viewpoint he expresses his conviction that animal research is of vital importance. Animal rights advocates who raid laboratories and propagandize against animal research, he asserts, are irrevocably damaging scientists' efforts to find cures for AIDS, cancer, and other life-threatening diseases.

As you read, consider the following questions:

1. The author describes several incidents of animal advocates disrupting medical research by damaging labs and freeing research animals. Do you agree with his opinion that these acts were unjustified and harmful to the advance of medicine? Explain.
2. Why does Hubbell consider many animal activists anti-human?
3. What overall impact on scientific research does the author say animal activism is having?

In the predawn hours of July 4, 1989, members of the Animal Liberation Front (ALF), an "animal rights" organization, broke into a laboratory at Texas Tech University in Lubbock. Their target: Prof. John Orem, a leading expert on sleep-disordered breathing.

The invaders vandalized Orem's equipment, breaking recorders, oscilloscopes and other instruments valued at some $70,000. They also stole five cats, halting his work in progress— work that could lead to an understanding of disorders such as Sudden Infant Death Syndrome (SIDS), or crib death, which kills over 5000 infants every year.

An organization known as People for the Ethical Treatment of Animals (PETA), which routinely issues press releases on ALF activities, quoted ALF claims that biomedical scientists are "animal-Nazis" and that Orem "abuses, mutilates and kills animals as part of the federal grant gravy train."

That was only the beginning of the campaign. A month later, on August 18, animal-rights activists held statewide demonstrations against Orem, picketing federal buildings in several Texas cities. The result: a flood of hate mail to the scientist and angry letters to the National Institutes of Health (NIH), which had awarded Orem more than $800,000 in grants. Finally PETA, quoting 16 "experts," filed a formal complaint with the NIH which called Orem's work "cruel" and without "scientific significance." The public had no way of knowing that none of the 16 had any expertise in sleep-disordered breathing or had ever been in Orem's lab.

NIH dispatched a team of authorities in physiology, neuroscience and pulmonary and veterinary medicine who, on September 18, reported back. Not only did they find the charges against Orem to be unfounded, but they judged him an exemplary researcher and his work "important and of the highest scientific quality."

Monkey Business

PETA first intruded on the public consciousness in 1981, during a notorious episode in Silver Spring, Md. That May, a personable college student named Alex Pacheco went to research psychologist Edward Taub for a job. Taub was studying monkeys under an NIH grant, searching for ways to help stroke victims regain use of paralyzed limbs. Pacheco said he was interested in gaining laboratory experience. Taub offered him a position as a volunteer, which Pacheco accepted.

Late that summer, Taub took a vacation, leaving his lab in the care of his assistants. As he was about to return to work on September 11, an assistant called. Police, armed with a search warrant, were confiscating the monkeys; there was also a crowd of reporters on hand.

To his amazement, Taub was charged with 119 counts of cruelty to animals—most based on information provided to the police by Alex Pacheco, who, it turned out, was one of PETA's founders.

After five years in the courts, Taub was finally cleared of all charges. Yet the animal-rights movement never ceased vilifying him, producing hate mail and death threats. Amid the controversy the NIH suspended and later terminated Taub's grant (essentially for not buying new cages, altering the ventilation system or providing regular visits by a veterinarian). Thorough investigations by the American Physiological Society and the Society for Neuroscience determined that, in the words of the latter, the NIH decision was "incommensurate with the deficiencies cited." Yet a program that could have benefited many of the 2.5 million Americans now living with the debilitating consequences of stroke came to a screeching halt.

Wiped out financially, Taub lost his laboratory, though the work of this gifted researcher had already helped rewrite accepted beliefs about the nervous system.

Early Anti-Vivisection Activism

The animal-rights movement has its roots in Europe, where anti-vivisectionists have held the biomedical research community under siege for years. In 1875, Britain's Sir George Duckett of the Society for the Abolition of Vivisection declared: "Vivisection is monstrous. Medical science has little to learn, and nothing can be gained by repetition of experiments on living animals."

This sentiment is endlessly parroted by contemporary "activists." It is patently false. Since Duckett's time, animal research has led to vaccines against diphtheria, polio, measles, mumps, whooping cough, rubella. It has meant eradication of smallpox, effective treatment for diabetes and control of infection with powerful antibiotics.

The cardiac pacemaker, microsurgery to reattach severed limbs, and heart, kidney, lung, liver and other transplants are all possible because of animal research. In the early 1960s, the cure rate for acute lymphocytic leukemia in a child was 4 percent. Today, because of animal research, the cure rate exceeds 70 percent. Since the turn of the century, animal research has helped increase our life-span by nearly 28 years. And now animal research is leading to dramatic progress against AIDS and Alzheimer's disease.

Animals themselves have benefited. We are now able to extend and improve the lives of our pets and farm animals through cataract surgery, open-heart surgery and cardiac pacemakers, and can immunize them against rabies, distemper, anthrax, tetanus and feline leukemia. Animal research is an unqualified success story.

We should see even more spectacular medical breakthroughs in the coming decades. But not if today's animal-rights movement has its way.

In the United States, the movement is spearheaded by PETA, whose leadership insists that animals are the moral equivalent of human beings. Any differentiation between people and animals constitutes "speciesism," as unethical as racism. Says PETA co-founder and director Ingrid Newkirk, "There really is no rational reason for saying a human being has special rights. . . . A rat is a pig is a dog is a boy." She compares the killing of chickens with the Nazi Holocaust. "Six million people died in concentration camps," she told the *Washington Post*, "but six billion broiler chickens will die this year in slaughterhouses."

Animals Are Essential

Laboratory animals are vital to the scientific process, and their welfare is of major concern to responsible scientists. As Robert White has argued in his article "The Facts About Animal Research," scientists feel that "valid work depends on clean, healthy research subjects that are not victims of physical or emotional stress." Except in rare (and widely publicized) cases, animals are not sadistically abused; in fact, a 1985 Department of Agriculture survey showed that only 6 percent of federally protected animals (excluding rats and mice) were allowed to feel pain as part of an experiment. Scientists have also acted to provide for the "psychological well-being" of their subjects, as mandated by amendments to the Animal Welfare Act of 1966, the original law governing animal care in laboratories. Chimpanzees at the Laboratory for Experimental Medicine and Surgery in Primates at New York University were given complex games and access to neighboring cages to prevent boredom and depression.

Scientists do acknowledge that alternatives to the use of animals have a potential in experimental research, but they also point out that these alternatives are not yet advanced enough to allow the research to continue without animal use.

Karl Biermann, *The Humanist*, July/August 1990.

Newkirk has been quoted as saying that meat-eating is "primitive, barbaric, arrogant," that humans have "grown like a cancer. We're the biggest blight on the face of the earth," and that if her father had a heart attack, "it would give me no solace at all to know his treatment was first tried on a dog."

The movement insists that animal research is irrelevant, that researchers simply refuse to move on to modern techniques.

"The movement's big buzzword is 'alternatives,' meaning animals can now be replaced by computers and tissue cultures," says Bessie Borwein, associate dean for research-medicine at the University of Western Ontario. "That is nonsense. You cannot study kidney transplantation or diarrhea or high blood pressure on a computer screen."

"A tissue culture cannot replicate a complex organ," echoes Frederick Goodwin, head of the U.S. Alcohol, Drug Abuse and Mental Health Administration (ADAMHA).

What do the nation's 570,000 physicians feel about animal research? A 1988 American Medical Association survey found that 97 percent of doctors support it, despite the animal-rights movement's propaganda to the contrary.

"Without animal research, medical science would come to a total standstill," says Dr. Lewis Thomas, best-selling author and scholar-in-residence at New York's Cornell University Medical College.

"As a human being and physician, I cannot conceive of telling parents their sick child will die because we cannot use all the tools at our disposal," says pioneering heart surgeon Dr. Michael E. DeBakey of Houston's Baylor College of Medicine. "How will they feel about a society that legislates the rights of animals above those of humans?"

"The power of today's medical practice is based on research—and that includes crucial research involving animals," adds Dr. Louis W. Sullivan, secretary of the U.S. Department of Health and Human Services.

Exploiting Public Sentiment

How then have the animal-rights activists achieved respectability? By exploiting the public's rightful concern for humane treatment of animals. ADAMHA's Goodwin explains: "They have gradually taken over highly respectable humane societies by using classic radical techniques: packing memberships and steering committees and electing directors. They have insidiously gained control of one group after another."

The average supporter has no idea that societies which traditionally promoted better treatment for animals, taught pet care, built shelters and cared for strays are now dedicated to ending the most effective kind of medical research. For example, the Humane Society of the United States (HSUS) insists it is not anti-vivisectionist; yet it has persistently stated that animal research is often unnecessary. It published an editorial by animal-rights proponent Tom Regan endorsing civil disobedience for the cause. Says Frederick A. King, director of the Yerkes Regional Primate Center of Emory University, "HSUS flies a false flag. It is part of the same group that has attempted to do severe damage to research."

PETA's chairman, Alex Pacheco, says that it is best to be "strategically assertive" in seeking reforms while never losing sight of the ultimate goal: "total abolition" of "animal exploitation." This strategy has worked. It has taken the research community about ten years to realize that it is not dealing with moderates. It is dealing with organizations like ALF, which since 1988 has been on the FBI's list of domestic terrorist organizations. And with Trans-Species Unlimited, which trumpets: "The liberation of animal life can only be achieved through the radical transformation of human consciousness and the overthrow of the existing power structures in which human and animal abuse are entrenched."

Liberation Activities

[But] consider some of the movement's "liberation activities":

• In the early hours of April 3, 1989, hooded animal-rights activists broke into four buildings at the University of Arizona at Tucson. They smashed expensive equipment, spray-painted messages such as "Scum" and "Nazis" and stole 1231 animals. They set fire to two of the four buildings.

ALF took credit for the destruction, the cost of which amounted to more than $200,000. Fifteen projects were disrupted. One example: 30 of the 1160 mice taken by ALF were infected with Cryptosporidium, a parasite that can cause severe intestinal disease in humans. The project's aim was to develop an effective disinfectant for Cryptosporidium-contaminated water. Now, not only is the work halted but researchers warn that, with less than expert handling, the stolen mice could spread cryptosporidiosis, which remains untreatable.

• On October 26, 1986, an ALF contingent broke into two facilities at the University of Oregon at Eugene. The equipment the intruders smashed and soaked with red paint included a $10,000 microscope, an electrocardiogram machine, an X-ray machine, an incubator and a sterilizer. At least 150 research animals were taken. As a result, more than a dozen projects were seriously delayed, including research by neuroscientist Barbara Gordon-Lickey on visual defects in newborns. An ALF statement called the neuroscientist a "butcher" and claimed that the animals had found new homes through "an intricate underground railroad network, much like the one used to transport fugitive slaves to the free states of the North in the last century."

Police caught up with one of the thieves: Roger Troen, 56, of Portland, Ore., a member of PETA. He was tried and convicted. PETA denied complicity, but Ingrid Newkirk said that PETA would pay Troen's legal expenses, including an appeal of his conviction. PETA then alleged to the NIH that the university was guilty of 12 counts of noncompliance with Public Health Service policy on humane care and use of laboratory animals.

Following a lengthy investigation, investigators found all PETA's charges groundless. "To the contrary," their report to the NIH stated, "evidence suggests a firm commitment to the appropriate care and use of laboratory animals."

But animal-rights extremists continued their campaign against Gordon-Lickey. They posted placards urging students not to take her courses because she tortured animals. As Nobel Laureate Dr. David H. Hubel of Harvard University, a pioneer in Gordon-Lickey's field, says, "Their tactics are clear. Work to increase the costs of research, and stop its progress with red tape and lawsuits."

• Dr. Herbert Pardes, president of the American Psychiatric Association, arrived in New York City in 1984 to take over as chairman of psychiatry at Columbia University. His office was in the New York State Psychiatric Institute, part of the Columbia Presbyterian Medical Center complex. Soon after, he noticed that people were handing out leaflets challenging the value of animal research. They picketed Dr. Pardes's home and sent him envelopes containing human feces.

Another Columbia scientist received a phone call on December 1, 1988, from someone who said, "We know where you live. How much insurance do you have?" A few mornings later, he found a pool of red paint in front of his house. On January 4, 1989, a guest cottage at his country home burned down.

Devastating Results

How effective has the animal-rights movement been? Very. Although recent polls reveal that more than 70 percent of Americans support animal research, about the same number believe the lie that medical researchers torture their animals.

According to ADAMHA's Frederick Goodwin, the movement has at its disposal at least $50 million annually, millions of which it dedicates to stopping biomedical research. It has been especially successful in pressuring state legislatures, as well as Congress, which in turn has pressured the federal health establishment. As a result, new regulations are demoralizing many scientists and driving up the cost of research. (For fiscal 1990, an estimated $1.5 billion—approximately 20 percent of the entire federal biomedical-research budget—may be needed to cover the costs of proposed regulation changes and increased security.)

At Stanford University, a costly security system has had to be installed and 24-hour guards hired to protect the animal-research facilities. As a consequence of the April 1989 raid at the University of Arizona at Tucson, the school must now spend $10,000 per week on security, money that otherwise could have been used for biomedical research.

Threats of violence to researchers and their families are having an effect as well. "It's hard to measure," says Charles R. McCarthy, director of the Office for Protection from Research Risks at the NIH. "But all of a sudden there is a hole in the kind of research being done."

In the past two years, for instance, there has been a 50- to 60-percent drop in the number of reports published by scientists using primates to study drug abuse. Reports on the use of primates to learn about severe depression have ended altogether.

And what of our future researchers? Between 1977 and 1987 there was a 28-percent drop in the number of college students graduating with degrees in biomedical science, and the growing influence of the animal-rights movement may add to that decline.

Stop the Fanatics

How are we to ensure that the animal-rights movement does not put an end to progress in medical research?

1. Don't swallow whole what the movement says about horrors in our biomedical-research laboratories. With rare exceptions, experimental animals are treated humanely. Biomedical researchers know that an animal in distress is simply not a good research subject. Researchers are embarked on an effort to alleviate misery, not cause it.

2. There are many humane societies that are truly concerned with animal welfare and oppose the animal-rights movement. They deserve your support. But before you contribute, make sure the society has not been taken over by animal-rights extremists. If you are not sure, contact iiFAR (incurably ill For Animal Research), P.O. Box 1873, Bridgeview, Ill. 60455. This organization is one of medical research's most effective allies.

3. Oppose legislation at local, state and federal levels that is designed to hamper biomedical research or price it out of business. Your representatives in government are lobbied by the animal-rights movement all the time. Let them know how *you* feel. . . .

If we want to defeat the killer diseases that still confront us— AIDS, Alzheimer's, cancer, heart disease and many others, the misguided fanatics of the animal-rights movement must be stopped.

"Over 100 years of animal research may have left our culture further behind in the search for wisdom than when the research started."

Animal Research Teaches Little

Roger E. Ulrich

A research professor at Western Michigan University in Kalamazoo, Roger E. Ulrich spent many years both as student and scientist engaged in animal research. In recent years, however, he has concluded that animal research adds little knowledge or wisdom to science, at least to the behavioral sciences in which he specializes. In the following viewpoint, he discusses this conclusion and argues that much animal research is done more out of unquestioned tradition than out of considered belief.

As you read, consider the following questions:

1. Near the beginning of this viewpoint, Ulrich quotes the great behaviorist B.F. Skinner. According to Ulrich, what assumptions in the Skinner quote explain the use of animals in research?
2. The author concludes that animal studies offer little knowledge to his field of study. In addition to viewing these studies as unhelpful, does he view them as harmful in any way? Explain.
3. List three things that ultimately led Ulrich to abandon animal research.

From Roger E. Ulrich, "Animal Research: A Psychological Ritual," *The Animals' Agenda*, May 1991. Reprinted with permission.

A fundamental assumption of the science of behavior is that studies of nonhuman animals can yield results that ultimately benefit humans. From Ivan Pavlov's dog conditioning experiments to the present day, animal researchers have generally assumed the view articulated by the late B.F. Skinner in 1953:

> We study the behavior of [nonhuman] animals because it is simpler. Basic processes are revealed more easily and can be recorded over longer periods of time. Our observations are not complicated by the social relations between subject and experimenter. Conditions may be better controlled. We may arrange genetic histories to control certain variables and special life histories to control others—for example, if we are interested in how an organism learns to see, we can raise an animal in darkness until the experiment is begun. We are also able to control current circumstances to an extent not easily realized in human behavior—for example, we can vary states of deprivation over wide ranges. These are advantages which should not be dismissed on the *a priori* contention that human behavior is inevitably set apart as a separate field.

The use of animals in behavioral studies is built upon such assumptions, and has evolved into a technology practiced mainly for the purpose of proving them.

Real Situations

A conflicting assumption, again skillfully articulated by Skinner in the novel *Walden Two*, is that ultimately there is no experiment other than a real situation:

> "Some of us feel that we can eventually find the answer in teaching and research," said Professor Burris.
>
> "In teaching, no. It's all right to stir people up, get them interested. That's better than nothing. But in the long run you're only passing the buck—if you see what I mean, sir." Rogers, the former student, paused in embarrassment.
>
> "For heavens sake, don't apologize," replied Professor Burris. "You can't hurt me there, that's not my Achilles heel."
>
> "What I mean, sir, is you've got to do the job yourself if it's ever going to be done, not just whip somebody else up to it. Maybe in your research you are getting close to the answer. I wouldn't know."
>
> "I'm afraid the answer is still a long way off," Burris demurred.
>
> "Well, that's what I mean, sir. It's a job for research, but not the kind you can do in a university, or a laboratory anywhere. I mean you've got to experiment and experiment with your own life, not just sit back in an ivory tower somewhere—as if your own life weren't all mixed up in it." Rogers stopped again.
>
> "Perhaps this was my Achilles heel," said Burris.

The contrived basic experimental laboratory that has evolved from Pavlov's work and the real-life application of knowledge are in fundamental conflict, a conflict increasingly evident from the failure of behavioral science to effectively respond to challenges including urban alienation, violent crime, child abuse, substance abuse, the continuing proliferation of age-old forms of mental illness, and what often seems to be a complete collapse of the elementary and secondary levels of our educational infrastructure. Effective responses in many cases have long since evolved, mainly at the clinical, police beat, or gradeschool classroom level; but at the academic level, where most of the federal mental health budget is spent, the emphasis is on research—mainly animal research—and the best minds in the behavioral field are continually directed into research, away from actual prevention and cure.

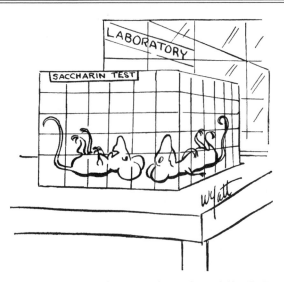

"I MUST SAY THE SEXUAL BEHAVIOR TESTS WERE
MORE FULFILLING THAN THIS ONE!"

In June of 1961 I completed my doctoral dissertation entitled "Reflexive Fighting in Response to Aversive Stimulation." The study, which involved shocking rats, showed that stereotyped fighting would occur between paired animals as a reflex-type reaction to pain prior to any specific conditioning. My paper was later published in the *Journal of the Experimental Analysis of Behavior.*

I was close to obtaining a Ph.D. in clinical/counseling psychology from Southern Illinois University, which was at that time trying to win American Psychological Association recognition for producing clinicians who were also scientists. Behind that effort was the inferiority complex felt by many clinical psychologists in the face of the American Medical Association and its psychiatrists. Only research with "quantifiable" data was acceptable to dissertation committees, whose basic behavioristic assumptions didn't allow for the contemplation of such variables as emotions, feelings, disgust, etc., nor for questioning why one was shocking rats in the first place.

Simultaneous with various animal research projects, I was also conducting studies with mental patients. My research with patients, however, was often looked upon by those who held radical behaviorist views as being too complex to allow for "clean data."

For me, the scientific attraction to animal research had, in the final analysis, little to do with a *demonstrable* relationship of research findings to the goal of "helping humans." In retrospect, I would say the main attraction to working with animals was, as Skinner proclaimed, "that we are able to control current circumstances to an extent not easily realized in human behavior." At any rate, after I earned my Ph.D., I joined the army of animal researchers who contended that we must conduct further experiments.

Laboratory aggression experiments provide a perfect example of basic research, in which the sequence of events leads from one animal experiment to the next, with each project following the preceding one as a direct consequence, and with each being essentially as irrelevant to solving real human problems as the one before. The fact that I have often sat behind closed doors with numerous colleagues who have agreed with this analysis is of little consequence to the animals still confined in laboratory cages around the world, because the true feelings of these professionals remain unexpressed.

Behind Closed Doors

Let us look beyond closed doors, however, at some additional data from the "contrived" research situation.

In 1948, a study was published by Neal E. Miller under the title, "Theory and experiment relating psychoanalytic displacement to stimulus-response generalization." It is a report of how Miller and his assistants trained rats to fight by removing the shock each time the animals approximated the fighting position. Fighting, they presumed, was an escape reaction, reinforced by the termination of electric shock. Our laboratory at Anna State Hospital was very much involved at the time in escape and avoidance research, and was especially concerned with the area of punishment. An attempt to replicate Miller's procedures, however, showed that fighting behavior could be elicited from paired rats with no training whatsoever. Here, now, was a perfect example showing not only that the Miller interpretation of results was incorrect, but also that a wrong-headed analysis was being used by people dedicated to using only "observable data.". . .

So it was that a trivial experiment (albeit not so to the rats), done by a well-known apologist for animal research, who had wrongly interpreted the results of his experiment, led to our shocking still more animals.

We, of course, went to the literature and somewhat unhappily discovered that what we had found had been found before by O'Kelly and Steckle in 1939. They titled their paper "A long enduring emotional response in the rat . . ." which no doubt it was, and which it continues to be to this day, inasmuch as rats are still being shocked to demonstrate the pain-aggression phenomenon.

When I told my Mennonite mother what we had found in my dissertation research, she said, "Well, we know that. Dad always told us to stay away from wounded animals on the farm because they might hurt you." Nevertheless, I entered into a ten-year period of dedicated analysis of the causes of aggression, hoping a better understanding of how to control human aggression would follow.

Controlling Aggression

In 1973 I finally came to the conclusion that if the control of human aggression was our goal, we were looking in the wrong place. I still was in no way enlightened in that area to the extent that I could offer meaningful advice to people who questioned me regarding aggression. Indeed, my own anger was often uncontrollable, despite my discoveries and laboratory knowledge. Thus one spring, in response to my department chairman's question, "What is the most innovative thing that you have done professionally during the past year?" I replied, "Dear Dave, I've finally stopped torturing animals."

As early as 1972 I had already stopped conducting traditional basic animal research, having demonstrated over and over in countless different ways what my grandpa had taught his children: when animals are hurt, they are more likely to be aggressive. Without fully realizing it at the time, I was divorcing myself from the vast armada of behavioral scientists who daily illustrate how animal research has become for them a self-reinforcing activity.

For ten years I had written on the topic of aggression; did research; traveled through Europe, Asia, Central and South America, and the U.S. talking on the topic; made movies about it; wrote grant requests to every local, state, and federal agency, private and public, that held even the remotest hope of giving money for my research. I helped design new strategies and new equipment for shocking anything that moved, and even observed children whom I had convinced to shock some rats and "watch what happens." More and more allegedly new discoveries were added to a voluminous literature, reprints of which I was collecting for a book and which now weigh close to 50 pounds. Studies leading to new studies, all involving countless animals, with the findings essentially irrelevant to people in that *at no time did the conditions under which the animals were studied equal the existing human conditions to which the generalizations were being "theoretically" transposed.* These permutations upon permutations conducted in the world's scientific laboratories with different species under countless different research conditions are nearly infinite.

The Real-Life Laboratory

Skinnerites, perhaps more than any other group of scientists, have called for the generalization of animal research findings into building a better tomorrow. Their persistent claim is that experimental analysis of animal behavior has enabled us to redesign human culture to enhance our chances of survival. But for me, as for Skinner's hero in *Walden Two*, faith in the ability of animal research to guarantee the continuance of humankind on earth is nothing less than pure superstition. Indeed, we are faced with a situation in which over 100 years of animal research may have left our culture further behind in the search for wisdom than when the research started.

In his book *Nature, Man and Woman*, Alan Watts summarizes:

> Based on the assumption that we had done wisely, and were still here and likely to remain, the human race had survived and seemed likely to go on surviving for perhaps more than a million years before the arrival of modern technology. We must on this premise assume that it had acted wisely thus far. We may argue that its life was not highly pleasant, but it is difficult to know what that means. The race was certainly pleased to go on living, for it did so.

> On the other hand, after a bare two centuries of industrial technology the prospects of human survival are being quite seriously questioned. It is not unlikely that we may propagate, eat and possibly blow ourselves off the planet.

As is the tradition in science, I will now call for further research. But this is the question we must explore: Can human society afford the assumption that the current level of animal research and sacrifice is worthy of our continued support?

My conclusion is no. The atrocities we persist in perpetrating within our laboratories, where scientists are paid to perform painful rituals on other lifeforms based on blind faith that human suffering might be driven away, should increasingly be questioned and discontinued. They are *not* reducing the suffering we so often feel and see around us in the real-life laboratory.

Our scientific addiction to animal research must be given up and replaced with the observation of natural phenomena. What B.F. Skinner said in his novel *Walden Two* about "the need for us to experiment with our own lives and not just sit back in an ivory tower somewhere—as if your own life weren't all mixed up in it," overshadows in importance every other point he ever made. If Skinner is to be remembered as an important voice in the history of science, it will be for his call to reconnect research with that which is relevant.

> *"No other options [except animal organs] exist for alleviating the scarcity in the supply of replacement parts."*

Humans Should Be Allowed to Receive Animal Organ Transplants

Arthur L. Caplan

In the following viewpoint, Arthur L. Caplan considers the question of xenografts, the transplantation of animal organs into human patients, a procedure still considered experimental. He believes that with the current scarcity of transplantable human organs, animals offer an excellent source for both "bridge" (temporary) and permanent organ transplantation. Head of the Center for Biomedical Ethics at the University of Minnesota in Minneapolis, Caplan is a prolific writer on biomedical topics.

As you read, consider the following questions:

1. What is the overriding factor, in Caplan's view, that justifies animal organ transplantation into humans?
2. Why does the author believe animal research is justified in the study of transplantation?
3. Does Caplan believe humans are inherently more valuable than animals? Paraphrase his view.

From Arthur L. Caplan, "Is Xenografting Morally Wrong?" *Transplantation Proceedings* 24 (April 1992): 722-27. Reprinted with permission.

It is tempting to think that a decision about whether or not it is immoral to use animals as sources for transplantable organs and tissues hinges only upon the question of whether or not it is ethical to kill them. But the ethics of xenografting involves more than an analysis of that question. And even the assessment of the morality of killing animals to obtain their parts to use in human beings is more complicated than it might at first glance appear to be.

To decide whether it is ethical to kill animals, a variety of subsidiary questions must be considered. Is it ethical to kill animals to obtain organs and tissues to save human lives or alleviate severe disability when it might not be ethical to kill them for food or sport? Why are animals being considered as sources of organs and tissues—do alternative methods for obtaining replacement parts for human beings exist? What sorts of animals would have to be killed, how would they be killed, and how would they be stored, handled, and treated prior to their deaths?

If it is possible to defend the killing of animals for xenografting then questions as to the morality of subjecting human beings to the risks, both physical and psychological, associated with xenografting must also be weighed. In undertaking a xenograft on a human subject the focus of moral concern ought not to be solely on the animal that will be killed.

Even for those who eat meat or hunt, it might well seem immoral to kill animals for their parts if alternative sources of replacement parts were or might soon be available. The moral acceptability of xenografting will for many, including the prospective recipients of animal parts, be contingent on the presumption that there is no other plausible alternative source of transplantable organs and tissues. Unfortunately, the scarcity that is behind the current interest in xenografting is all too real.

Inadequate Human Organ Supply

Why pursue xenografting? The supply of organs and tissues available from human cadaveric sources for transplantation in the United States and other nations is entirely inadequate. Many children and adults die or remain disabled due to the shortage of transplantable organs and tissues. Unless some solution is found to the problem of scarcity, the plight of those in need of organs and tissues will only grow worse and the numbers who die solely for want of an organ will continue to grow.

More than one-third of those now awaiting liver transplants die for want of a donor organ. Well over one-half of all children born with fatal, congenital deformities of the heart or liver die without a transplant due to the shortage of organs. The percentage of those who die while waiting would actually be higher if all potential candidates were on waiting lists.

Some Americans are not referred for transplants because they cannot afford them. If those with organ failure from economically underdeveloped nations were wait-listed at North American and European transplant centers, the percentage of those who die while awaiting a transplant would be much larger.

More than 150,000 Americans with kidney failure are kept alive by renal dialysis. The cost for this treatment exceeded five billion dollars in 1988. It would be far cheaper and, from the patient perspective as to the quality of life, far more desirable to treat kidney failure by means of transplants. But, there are simply not enough cadaveric kidneys for all who desire and could benefit from a transplant.

The supply of cadaveric organs for pancreas, small intestine, lung, heart-lung transplants for those dying of a wide variety of diseases affecting these organs is not adequate. The same story holds for bone, ligament, dural matter, heart valves, and skin. Moreover, demand for the limited supply of organs and tissues is increasing as more and more medical centers become capable of offering this form of surgery and as techniques for managing rejection and infection improve.

The shortage of organs and tissues for transplantation has led researchers to pursue a variety of alternatives in order to bridge the gap between supply and demand. Some suggest changing existing public policies governing cadaveric procurement. Others focus on locating alternatives to human cadaveric organs. . . .

It is the plight of those dying of end-stage diseases for want of donor organs from both living and cadaveric human sources that has led a number of research groups to explore the option of using animals as the source of transplantable organs and tissues. Transplant researchers at Loma Linda, the University of Pittsburgh, Stanford, Columbia, and Minnesota as well as in England, China, Belgium, Sweden, Japan, and France, among other countries, are conducting research on xenografting organs and tissues. Some are exploring the feasibility of primate to human transplants. Others are pursuing lines of research that would allow them to utilize animals other than primates as sources.

It is scarcity that grounds the moral case for thinking about animals as sources of organs and tissues. In light of current and potential demand, no other options exist for alleviating the scarcity in the supply of replacement parts. . . .

Ethical Problems with the Xenograft Option

If it is true that the case for pursuing xenografting is a persuasive one then the question of whether xenografting is morally wrong shifts to an analysis of which animals will be used, how they will be kept and killed, and the risks and dangers involved for potential human recipients. Xenografting is still evolving so the ethical issues must be considered under two broad headings; issues associated with basic and clinical experimentation and, if this proves successful, those that would then be associated with the widespread use of xenografts as therapies.

In thinking about the ethics of research on xenografting a couple of assumptions can safely be made. The number and type of animals used will be very much a function of cost, prior knowledge of the species, inbred characteristics, ease in handling, and availability. Gorillas are not going to be used in research simply because there are too few of them and they are unlikely to make compliant subjects. Rats and mice will dominate the early stages of research (as they already do) because they are relatively well understood, special-purpose bred, and cheap to acquire and maintain. Few primates will be used for basic or clinical research simply because they are too scarce, too expensive, and too complex to permit controlled study for most experimental purposes.

Cross-Species Testing

Even if the number of animals to be used is relatively small, the question still must be faced as to whether it is ethical to use animal models involving species such as rats, chickens, sheep, pigs, monkeys, baboons, and chimps in order to study the feasibility of cross-species xenografting. In part, the answer to this question pivots on whether or not there are plausible alternative models to the use of animals for exploring the two critical steps required for successful xenografting—overcoming immunologic rejection and achieving long-term physiologic function in an organ or tissue.

To some extent, immunologic problems can be examined without killing primates or higher animals by using lower animals or cellular models. But there would not appear to be any viable alternatives or nonhuman substitutes available for understanding the processes involved in rejection. At best it may be possible to utilize animals that have fewer cognitive and intellectual capacities for most forms of basic research with respect to understanding the immunology of xenografting.

When research gets closer to the clinical stage especially when it becomes possible to examine the extent to which xenografted organs and tissues can function post-transplant, it will be necessary to use some animals as donors and recipients that are closely related to human beings. If, in light of the scarcity of human organs, it is ethical to pursue the option of xenografting, then, it would be unethical to subject human beings to any form of xenografting that has not undergone a prior demonstration of both immunologic and physiologic feasibility in animals closely analogous to humans.

226

The use of animals analogous to humans for basic research on xenografting means that some form of primates must be used both as donors and as recipients. Is it ethical to kill primates, even if only a small number, to demonstrate the feasibility of xenografting in human beings? . . .

The debate about the morality of killing a primate of some sort to advance human interests by saving human lives then hinges on empirical facts about what particular species of primates can or cannot do in comparison to what humans are capable of doing.

Humanity's Needs Are Primary

Because of the clear distinction drawn between the nature of man and animals, if there is conflict between the well-being of one and the other then man's well-being must automatically come first. The application of such a philosophical approach to the problem of animal experimentation for medical need is helpful in a situation where emotions again give us opposing signals: a desire to cure human disease and a desire not to harm animals. [This] approach clearly justifies the pain of animals in the service of relieving the pain of man. However, it would require that animal experimentation was done in the kindest way possible to help promote kindness towards man in the world.

John Martin, *Journal of Medical Ethics*, 1990.

It is indisputable that there are some differences in the capacities and abilities of humans and primates. Chimps can sign but humans have much more to say. Gorillas seem to reason but humans have calculus, novels, and quantum theory. Humans are capable of a much broader range of behavior and intellectual functioning then are any specific primate species.

Many who would protest the use of primates in xenografting research are keen to illustrate that primates possess many of the properties and abilities that are found to contribute moral standing to humans. The fact that one species or another of primate is capable of some degree of intellectual or behavioral ability that seems worthy of moral respect when manifest by humans does not mean that human beings are the moral equivalents of primates. It is one thing to argue that primates ought to have moral standing. It is a very different matter to argue that humans and primates are morally equivalent. One can grant that primates deserve moral consideration without conceding that, on average, the death of a human being is of greater moral significance than is the death of a baboon, a green monkey, or a chimpanzee.

Xenografting involving primates can be morally justified on the grounds that, in general, human beings possess capacities and abilities that confer more moral value upon them than do primates. This is not "speciesism" but, rather, a claim of comparative worth that is based on important empirical differences between two classes or sets of creatures.

Perhaps there are empirical reasons to support the claim that it is worth killing primates for humans on the grounds that as groups humans have properties that confer greater moral worth and standing upon them than do other animal species. Human beings are after all moral agents while, at most, animals, even primates, are moral subjects.

Even conceding this point, there is still a problem when it comes time to kill a baboon and a chimp to see if xenografting between them is possible. Critics might ask whether scientists would be willing to kill a retarded child or an adult in a permanent vegetative state in the service of the same scientific goal? It is indisputable that human beings have on average more capacities and abilities than do animals. But there are some individual animals, many of them primates, that have more capacities and abilities than certain individual human beings who lack them due to congenital disorders or as the result of disease or injury. If it is argued that we ought to use animals instead of humans to assess the feasibility of xenografting because humans are more highly developed in terms of intellectual and emotional capacities, capacities that make a moral difference in that they are the basis for moral agency, then why should we not use a severely retarded child instead of a bright chimp or gorilla as subjects in basic or clinical research? . . .

Why Not Children?

One line of response is to simply say that we are powerful and the primates are less, therefore they must yield to human purposes if we choose to experiment upon them rather than retarded children. This line of response sounds rather far removed from the kinds of arguments we expect to be mustered in the name of morality. A more promising line of attack on the view that humans and primates or other animals are morally equivalent is to examine a bit more closely why it is that we would not want to use a retarded child instead of a chimp in basic research.

Two reasons might be given for picking a chimp instead of a human being with limited or damaged capacities. We might decide not to use a human being who has lost his or her capacities and abilities out of respect for their former existence. If the person makes a conscious decision to allow his or her body to be used for scientific research prior to having become comatose or brain dead then perhaps those wishes should be honored. If no such advance notice has been given then we ought not to presume anything about what they would have wanted and should forego any involvement in medical research generally and xenografting in particular on the grounds that this is what is demanded out of respect for the persons they once were.

However, severely retarded children or those born with devastating conditions such as anencephaly have never had the capacities and abilities that confer a greater moral standing on humans as compared with animals. Should they be used as the first donors and recipients in xenografting research instead of primates?

The reason they should not has nothing to do with the properties, capacities, and abilities of children or infants who lack and have always lacked significant degrees of intellectual and cognitive function. The reason they should not be used is because of the impact using them would have upon other human beings, especially their parents and relatives. A severely retarded child can still be the object of much love, attention, and devotion from his or her parents. These feelings and the abilities and capacities that generate them are deserving of moral respect. I do not believe animals including primates are capable of such feelings.

Parental Choices

If a human mother were to learn that her severely retarded son had been used in lethal xenografting research she would mourn this fact for the rest of her days. A baboon, monkey, or orangutan would not. The difference counts in terms of whether it is a monkey or a retarded human being who is selected as a subject in xenografting research.

It may be that parents would want to volunteer their child's organ or tissue for research or they might wish to have their baby with anencephaly serve as the first recipient of an animal organ or tissue. It may be necessary to honor such a choice. Whatever public policies are created to govern our actions toward severely retarded children or babies born with most of their brain missing, these are policies that are meant to be respectful of the sensibilities and interests of other human beings. They do not find their source in some inherent property of the anencephalic infant. It is in the relationships with others, both family and strangers, that the moral worth and standing of these children are grounded.

The case for using animals, even primates, before using a human being with severely limited abilities and capacities is based on the relationships that exist among human beings, which do not have parallels in the animal kingdom. These relationships, such as love, loyalty, empathy, sympathy, family-feeling, protectiveness, shame, community-mindedness, a sense of history, and a sense of responsibility, which ground many moral duties and set the backdrop for distinguishing virtuous conduct and character, do not, despite the sociality of some species, appear to exist among animals.

If animals are to be used then what sorts of guidelines should animal care and use committees or other review bodies follow in reviewing basic research proposals? These committees must ensure that basic research is designed in such a fashion as to minimize the need for animal subjects while maximizing the opportunity to obtain generalizable knowledge. They must also ensure that the animals used are kept in optimal conditions and are handled humanely and killed without pain. These steps will be necessary in order to both respect the moral standing of the animals and to maximize the chance for generating useful knowledge from the use of these animals in research. . . .

What about systematically breeding, raising, and killing animals for their parts on a large scale? Is it moral to systematically farm and kill animals for spare parts for humans? Would it be right to systematically farm and kill animals for spare parts for other animals, say companion animals?

One response to the issue of breeding and raising animals in order to have a regular supply of organs for xenografting is to argue that this practice does not raise any new or special moral issues since huge numbers of animals are currently bred, raised, and killed solely for consumption. However, animals raised for food are often raised under inhumane and brutal conditions. Nor is there much consideration given to the techniques involved in their slaughter. Animals that are to be used to generate a constant source of organs and tissues for transplant must be raised under conditions that would ensure the healthiest possible animals. The moral obligation to potential recipients would seem to require that systematic farming of animals only be permitted under the most humane circumstances.

Interestingly the issue of whether it is morally permissible to systematically breed, raise, and kill animals to obtain their parts does not raise the same issues of moral equivalence between animals and humans that arise with respect to basic and clinical research. It would obviously be immoral to breed, raise, and kill humans for their parts.

The availability of animal organs for transplant on a therapeutic basis is likely to become a matter of economics. The economics of this sort of animal breeding must take into account the costs of creating the healthiest possible animals and the most painless modes of killing. However, should xenografting evolve to the point of therapy, those who perform xenografts must also strive to ensure that access to transplants is equitable.

"We should reject . . . solving the problem of organ shortage by maintaining colonies of animals at the ready for transplantation on demand. "

Humans Should Not Be Allowed to Receive Animal Organs

James Lindemann Nelson

Some experts justify the use of animal organs for human implantation on the grounds that animals have lesser intellects than humans do. In the following viewpoint, James Lindemann Nelson questions this use of animal organs. Nelson points out that some humans—anencephalic infants and severely retarded persons, for example—have lesser intellects than many animals. Yet society would not think of using these humans in the same ways it uses animals. Nelson suggests that there are better ways to try to save lives than by killing animals for their organs. Nelson is an associate for ethical studies at the Hastings Center, a biomedical think tank in Briarcliff Manor, New York.

As you read, consider the following questions:

1. What comparison does Nelson make between abortion and the use of animals in medical research?
2. What is the author's basic repugnance against the use of animals for organ transplantation purposes?
3. What does Nelson suggest as a better way to deal with the present transplantable organ shortage?

James Lindemann Nelson, "Transplantation Through a Glass Darkly," *Hastings Center Report* 22 (September/October 1992): 6-8, © The Hastings Center. Reproduced by permission.

Bioethical problems take many different forms, and fascinate many different kinds of people. Physicians and philosophers, lawyers and theologians, policy analysts and talk show hosts are all drawn by the blend of practical urgency and moral complexity that characterize these issues.

But there seem to be only two kinds of bioethical problems that typically pull into their orbits not only theorists and practitioners, but pickets and protesters as well. When it comes to the treatment of fetuses and animals, people take to the streets. On the same day that demonstrators on both sides of the abortion issue lamented the Supreme Court's decision in *Casey*, representatives of PETA (People for the Ethical Treatment of Animals) gathered at the University of Pittsburgh to protest the implantation of a baboon's liver in a thirty-five-year-old man—the father of two children—whose own liver had been destroyed by hepatitis B virus [HBV].

There is, of course, a big difference in the way the disputes are perceived: abortion's bona fides as a central ethical issue are well established, but despite an upsurge of interest among ethicists over the past decade and a half, concern about animals still seems a bit quirky, too exclusively the domain of zealots who maintain the moral equality of all species, and thereby mark themselves as fundamentally out of sympathy with our basic ethical traditions. Here I try to pull moral consideration of nonhumans closer to the ethical center, arguing that thinking about the fate of nonhumans at our hands shares with abortion—indeed, with many of our culture's most difficult moral issues—a fundamental problem: we don't really know what we are talking about. More concretely, we're at a loss to say what it is about baboons that makes their livers fair game, when we wouldn't dare take vital organs from those of our own species whose abilities to live rich, full lives are no greater than those of the nonhumans we seem so willing to prey upon. Unless we're able to isolate and defend the relevant moral distinction, we should reject the seductive image of solving the problem of organ shortage by maintaining colonies of animals at the ready for transplantation on demand.

Moral Outliers

Public protest about abortion is not galvanized by concern about the quality of informed consent, or its impact on the doctor-patient relationship. What *does* lie at the center of the dispute is an absolutely crucial kind of ignorance. As a society, we don't know what fetuses are, and, in an important sense, we don't know what pregnant women are either. Are fetuses babies or tissue? Are pregnant women mothers bound by special duties to their unborn children, or independent adults exercising their right to make important self-regarding decisions under the protection of a mantle of privacy? Because we don't know these things, and they matter so much, we have a hard time imagining what responsible compromise might really be like.

And what gets people out into the streets in response to a daring attempt to rescue from certain death a young father of two? What, for that matter, causes medical research advocacy organizations to spend large amounts of money, not on research, but on full-page ads in the *New York Times* defending what scientists do? Is it concerns about justice in the allocation of medical resources? Doubts about the "courage to fail" ethos? Misgivings centered around the independence of IRB review? Surely not. The ground of protest and counterprotest is a similar kind of ignorance about the fundamental terms of the relevant moral discourse: we don't know what animals are, either. We treat them as if they were morally protean; we mold them unto anything from much-loved companions and symbols of virtue to mere machines for making food and instruments for scientific research.

The Edges of Moral Concern

Our ignorance as a society about these dark corners of our moral commitments, our lack of consensus about where outliers really fit, is extremely divisive when coupled with individual assurance that there is in fact available knowledge about these matters, that the answers are of surpassing importance, and that there is something suspicious, if not downright evil, about the people who don't get it. While such conclusions cripple civility, and should of course be resisted, our history should be making us nervous. We have so often gotten matters of who counts morally just flatly wrong, and have exacted horrible prices from those shuffled unjustly to the margins of our moral concern.

What fetuses are has at least received a thorough airing in the bioethics literature. Gravid women we still find quite puzzling apparently, as witness current concerns about "forced cesareans" and "maternal-fetal conflict," but at least there is an awareness that getting clear about the moral character of pregnancy is a key to understanding the morality of pregnancy terminations. But despite their ubiquity in medical research and practice, determining what animals are is not thought of as a paradigmatic bioethics issue. Yet seeing animals clearly is likely to be at least as difficult as the analogous tasks for fetuses and pregnant women. After all, we have a strong stake in the presumption that nonhumans are things whose moral status is at our discretion: the looser we can keep the moral constraints, the freer we are to do as we like with these extremely useful creatures. Further, there is a sense in which animals really are protean. Human beings are animals; so are protozoa. Drawing some moral distinctions is inescapable when facing such a range, and if there's to be a bright line between entities that really matter and those that don't, the human species may very well seem a reasonable place to draw it.

Choosing this line may appear suspiciously self-serving. Yet, at least at first glance, it looks as though there really could be something ethically serious to be said for us. We don't have to rely on the brute fact that we're got all the power; this is a comfort, as "might makes right" has a dubious history as a basis for moral distinctions. Nor do we have to resort to the bare fact of our common species membership—again, all to the good, as such purely biological bases for moral categorization also have a simply horrifying pedigree. Further, we can avoid invoking the soul as a sort of special moral talisman whose possession elevates us above all others: purely metaphysical entities aren't much use when we're trying to do ethics with an eye to public policy in a pluralistic society. Besides, imagine what we would do if someone were to argue that the subjugation of women was justified on the grounds that all and only men possess "schmouls," an empirically undetectable entity that inexplicably gives them extra moral worth.

Transplants Distract from Better Treatments

Chronic hepatitis is a serious disease. It kills about 6,000 Americans every year. While hepatitis often passes on its own with no treatment, for a fraction of patients the disease becomes chronic and debilitating.

Even so, the baboon-to-human liver transplants performed by . . . experimenters are not the answer. First of all, this is an experiment, not a treatment. That means the commitment of millions of dollars and many lives, both human and animal, with no clear likelihood of success. And it means the inevitable sacrifice of researchers' time and resources that are needed for other better treatments. . . .

Cross-species transplants have been a dream of some researchers for years—an impossible biological barrier to be assaulted with a steady surgical hand and some good immunosuppressant drugs. In chasing that peculiar surgical vision, realistic medical treatments may well be lost. And that is the real tragedy.

Neal D. Barnard, *San Diego Union-Tribune*, January 13, 1993.

The distinction we wish to draw between humans and the rest of creation seems much more respectable than distinctions based on might, on species, or on sectarian metaphysics. One could say that the appeal to such things as the range and power of the human intellect, the complexity and depth of our interpersonal relationships, our passions, both personal and aesthetic, our sense of morality, and of tragedy makes good sense. If these abilities and vulnerabilities don't matter morally, it's hard to imagine what would.

But if these are the characteristics that matter morally, it is not only baboons who lack them; not all of us humans have them either. Many humans have lost, or will never have, powerful intellects, deep relationships, rich passions, or the intimations of mortality. Think of the profoundly mentally ill, the comatose, and those who have sustained severe brain injuries. While such humans are themselves instances of tragedy, they have no sense of what tragedy is.

Despite this sad fact, our convictions about the importance of simply being human are so strong that we hesitate to use organs from newborns with anencephaly, a condition incompatible with either sensation or life. Given this hesitation, one can imagine the response if a leading transplant surgeon were to call for the maintenance of colonies of mentally handicapped orphans, to be well cared for until needed, but whose organs would then be "humanely" harvested for use in dying but otherwise "normal" people—infants with hypoplastic left heart syndrome, young fathers with HVB. Yet this scenario—with baboons and other primates substituting for handicapped orphans—is precisely what some transplant surgeons have been advocating since at least the 1960s, and is quite explicitly part of the agenda underlying the recent effort in Pittsburgh. If we are morally repulsed by a call to use handicapped orphans, but are eager to see whether colonies of baboons mightn't become a solution to our endemic lack of transplantable organs, it surely behooves us to have a good answer to the question, "What's so different about the two kinds of creature?"

Costs and Benefits of Xenografting

Perhaps there is a good answer to that question—a difference, or set of overlapping differences, that will end up ethically supporting our practice. Perhaps we could, without arbitrary prejudice, keep all mentally handicapped humans, no matter how damaged or how alone in the world they might be, in the ethical family, so to speak. Perhaps it's appropriate to see all nonhumans, no matter how intelligent or complex their lives might be, as largely discretionary items, to be cast into the outer darkness if anything approaching a serious purpose seems to demand it. Or perhaps the real moral of the story here is that it is not baboons we should respect more, but humans who are their emotional and intellectual peers we should respect less; consider the research and therapeutic bonanza *that* would yield! But defending either of these conclusions would take a powerful argument, and there's very little evidence that any of the people most enthusiastically thumping the tub for more and better xenotransplantation have come up with reasons of the kind that are needed. Typically, their strategy is simply to point to the human cost of not pushing the xenograft agenda—the "three people who die every day waiting for a necessary organ" argument—without any serious attempt to balance that cost against the debit incurred to the victims of those grafts. Nor do we see much effort to set the xenograft strategy against the costs and benefits incurred by trying to enforce the required request laws that are already on the books, or to enact "presumed consent" or "routine retrieval" policies for organ procurement.

Discernment in the Dark

This, of course, returns us to our original problem: we don't even know how to begin that balancing act, and it seems that we aren't very keen on learning. A simple reliance on our moral intuitions isn't enough. As the history of medical research in the nineteenth and even twentieth century reveals, we have been more than willing to subject those who were "clearly less valuable" to the rigors of research—only then, the ones who were obviously less valuable were Jewish, or people of color. Our gut instincts simply aren't good enough as reliable moral guides when we're dealing with those whom we've pushed to the margin of moral discourse The question is not whether we're generally able to move deftly within our ordinary understanding of morality, but whether, when it comes to the moral outliers, that ordinary understanding itself is adequate

Cross-species transplantation crystallizes a certain kind of moral conflict between humans and other animals—perhaps too sharply. Pitting the life of the father of two against that of a baboon is sure to strike most of us as no contest. The glare of the contrast distracts us from such realities as the fact that, at the point of decisionmaking, the animal's death buys only a chance, not a guarantee, or that the outcome of acting is not always better than the outcome of refraining, even when death is inevitable if we stay our hand. If we reflect about our moral duties and liberties more broadly, it may strike us that we are apparently quite comfortable allowing many tragic deaths to occur daily, when what it would take to stop them is not the life of an intelligent animal, but merely the cost of drinks after work.

On the other hand, if we do refuse to take the baboon's life in an effort to save the human's out of a sense that the moral parity between baboons and mentally handicapped humans leaves us no other option, then we need to ask what else that sense of parity implies. The animal who provided the liver in the Pittsburgh case was at least killed in an effort to save the life of an identifiable person. But most of what we do with the lives of animals is—at best—only distantly related to the lives and health of people in general. If it is wrong to kill a baboon to try to save a man's life, is it wrong to kill a pig because sausages taste so good? To kill a kid to make elegant gloves? Critics of xenograft whose main concern is with the "sacrificed" animal may find it relatively easy to adopt vegan diets and eschew wearing leather. But do they really advocate that ill people begin a wholesale boycott of a medical system in which the training and research leading up to its quite standard offerings are, as it were, drenched in the blood of nonhumans?

The implications of all this for the development of xenograft and the creation of "donor" colonies are comparatively clear. There are numerous ways in which we might strive to save and enhance lives, including many that are more efficient than killing animals who resemble us in no small degree—ways that do not burden us by reinforcing our commitment to moral positions we do not fully understand, and may not be able to maintain. If we feel morally constrained to continue organ transplantation as an important way of saving and enhancing human lives, we ought not to try to respond to that moral challenge with the technological fix of a better antirejection drug that will allow us to use nonhumans as organ sources, but rather by figuring out better ways to engage the altruism of the human community, until at last it strikes us all as mighty peculiar that anyone would want to hang on to her organs after death, when she has no conceivable use for them.

We ought to drop xenograft research and therapy, investing the resources of human effort, ingenuity, and money it consumes elsewhere. We don't now know what the judgment of history regarding our relationship with nonhumans will be, but there's no reason to be sanguine about it. What this uncertainty says for our overall relationship with animals may still be a matter for debate, but there's no compelling need to make matters any worse.

"The power to control the genetic engineering of animals lies in our hands."

Genetic Research on Animals Will Benefit Humanity

Caroline Murphy

In the following viewpoint, Caroline Murphy asserts that genetic engineering is here to stay and that it can make many positive contributions to humanity. But, she cautions, thoughtful decisions must be made to keep the science beneficial. Murphy, education officer for the Royal Society for the Prevention of Cruelty to Animals in England, holds advanced degrees in medicine, biology, and genetics.

As you read, consider the following questions:

1. According to the author, why is the idea of genetic engineering frightening to so many people?
2. List three of the positive contributions Murphy suggests the genetic engineering of animals can offer humankind.
3. Why does Murphy call genetic experimentation a Pandora's box? Does she think this Pandora's box must be kept closed? Explain.

Excerpted from Caroline Murphy, "Genetically Engineered Animals." In *The Bio-Revolution*, edited by Peter Wheale and Ruth McNally, published in 1990 by Pluto Press, London. Reprinted with permission.

Making animals that are a mixture of different species is not a new idea, but it is a new reality. One consequence of this is that there is a common ground that we all share when we start thinking about the type of genetic engineering that we call the transgenic manipulation of animals. Here I describe briefly what transgenic manipulation is, and point out some implications which may be both reassuring and disconcerting.

For many people, the transgenic manipulation of animals is a very frightening concept. The reason why we should find this application of modern genetics so disturbing lies at least partly in our cultural heritage. The fantasy of animals with a mix of characteristics of various species can be found in the culture of many ancient, and not so ancient, civilisations. When trying to decide what our reactions to transgenic animals should be we must be aware that many of us will have seen, or chosen not to see, feature films about mad scientists who have shut themselves away from the world and set about producing half-human, half-beast monsters. Mary Shelley's *Frankenstein* nightmare has produced many abiding cultural images and exposed deep-seated fears about the consequences of mankind's interference with nature. When we look at transgenic animals we must be aware that our reactions to them are unlikely to be based on the rational analysis of facts ably presented; the nightmare images from past fantasies are too likely to escape from the Pandora's Box of our imagination and distort our vision.

Transgenic Manipulation

Transgenic manipulation is a type of genetic engineering. It can loosely be described as taking genes from one organism and inserting them into the genetic material of another. A gene is a length, or a series of lengths, of DNA which carries the code for the sequence of amino acids that make up a protein. Every different protein has a unique amino acid sequence: that sequence is coded for in a gene. The genes lie interspersed with regulatory DNA in a fixed order along the chromosomes. There are gene-bearing chromosomes in the nuclei of all actively dividing cells and they are large enough to be seen under a light-microscope in a dividing cell nucleus. A gene is too small to see with the light-microscope, but banding patterns, generated by staining techniques, help us to 'map' the location of genes on chromosomes fairly accurately. For example, using a variety of gene mapping techniques, we have identified that the gene for the blood protein alpha globin is, in humans, on chromosome 16. In transgenic manipulation, a gene from one species relocates permanently—the scientists hope—into one of the chromosomes of another species.

When a sperm fertilises an egg, the chromosomes of the

mother and father pair up to produce the unique genetic characteristics of the offspring. Today's genetic engineering of transgenic animals involves the insertion of relatively small amounts of DNA. The amount of foreign DNA inserted into the chromosomes is so small that it does not interfere with this chromosome pairing process. Therefore transgenic animals are able to interbreed with each other and with other (non-transgenic) members of their species. It is hoped that the foreign gene, like any other gene, is passed on to about half the offspring. The normal transmission of half of each parent's genes to each offspring can apply to transgenic animals so successfully that, by normal mating of two different transgenics, young are born carrying both transgenes.

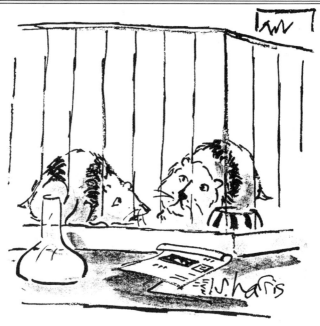

"As I understand it, our reactions were so remarkable, *we're* getting the Nobel prize."

The first experiments with transgenic manipulation were undertaken with bacteria and viruses. The commercial application of this work offers possibilities to people and animals. Bacteria carrying the gene for making the human insulin protein have already been produced. These bacteria have been cultured to produce commercial quantities of human insulin for use in place of insulin derived from pig or cow pancreases. However, many patients find it harder to control their diabetes using the new genetically engineered human insulin than using the insulins extracted from pigs or cows.

Nowadays transgenic plants and animals are being created in the laboratory. If wheat could be genetically engineered to fix nitrogen from the air (as the legumes can, naturally), wildlife could benefit from reduced run-off from nitrogenous fertilisers into streams and rivers.

But what about the genetic engineering of animals? The science magazine *Nature* introduced the reality of transgenic animals to the world with a spectacular front cover (*Nature* 1982). The cover depicted two apparently perfectly healthy mice; one of normal size, together with a 'giant' transgenic sibling with the growth hormone gene of a rat in every cell of its body. This 'giant' mouse was one of only seven transgenics produced from 170 specially treated egg cells. The researchers who had genetically engineered these transgenic mice nonetheless recognised that: 'the implicit possibility is to use this technology to stimulate the rapid growth of commercially valuable animals. Benefit would presumably come from a shorter production time and possibly from increased efficiency of food utilisation'.

The pigs carrying human growth hormone genes produced by USDA [United States Department of Agriculture] scientists at Beltsville in Maryland, USA, were among the first and most widely publicised transgenic animals. These pigs expressed high levels of growth hormone and developed severe arthritic deformities, probably as result of the regulatory gene sequence attached to the human growth hormone gene.

Applications

There are three main types of genetic engineering of vertebrates being carried out at the moment. These are the production of animal disease models for use in medical research; the production of pharmaceutically useful human proteins in animals, and the production of 'improved' agricultural animals. Each of these applications of genetic engineering may have both a positive and a negative side. The sheep which produce Factor IX in their milk are fit and healthy. Factor IX is the human blood-clotting factor missing in a type of haemophilia called 'Christmas disease'. If sheep could similarly be genetically engineered so that they lactate Factor VIII the absence of which is the most common cause of haemophilia, haemophiliacs the world over could benefit.

Much valuable grazing land in Africa cannot be used by farmers because of tsetse flies which carry various trypanosome parasites that cause diseases in cattle and humans, notably 'sleeping-sickness'. If cows could be genetically engineered to be resistant to these parasites, the farmers would be able to graze more land. In the short term, this might be good for the farmers and their stock, but the wild animals which are already resistant to 'sleeping-sickness' would be deprived of undisturbed grazing land, and their numbers would be bound to fall further as they were pushed to more marginal land.

The first patented mouse had a human cancer gene inserted into its genome so that it could act as a more 'accurate' model of human cancer than the mice that were already used. These patented mice are already on the market and were first imported into the UK in the spring of 1989. . . .

Poultry producers, worried about the spread of infectious disease through the large flocks of intensively reared birds, are very interested in the prospect of transgenic birds resistant to highly infectious viral infections, such as 'Newcastle Disease' (avian influenza). Those concerned about the birds' welfare question the humaneness of battery production systems. 'The Trojan horse' of disease resistance may provide a means whereby genetic engineers can design animals to cope with conditions that no animal, genetically engineered or not, should be expected to endure.

Another proposal is the production of cows which do not metabolise and break down their naturally produced growth hormone protein—bovine somatotropin (BST). Such cows could be genetically engineered so that they contain extra copies of the BST gene. The consequence of this would be cows, possibly patentable, producing high milk yields due to abnormal levels of their own BST. . . .

I have drawn attention to the important cultural role of mythical beasts—human-animal and animal-animal hybrids—in providing us all with nightmarish preconceptions about the crossing of species barriers. Scientists and welfarists alike must guard the Pandora's Box of our imaginations in assessing future realities. The Pandora's Box of the human imagination tempts scientists to out-do Doctor Frankenstein, and tempts welfarists to shut the lid on what may offer a cornucopia of opportunities. We must neither assume that all genetic engineering is evil, nor be seduced into thinking that the bright light of science can offer only progress. The genetic engineering of animals is here to stay. It offers both possibilities and problems that we must address intelligently. While the mythical 'transgenic' creatures of the past were thought to control our destiny, the power to control the genetic engineering of animals lies in our hands. We must ensure that we regulate and control this new technique to the benefit of both ourselves and other animals.

"The mind that views animals as pieces of coded genetic information to be manipulated and exploited at will is the mind that would view human beings in a similar way."

Genetic Research on Animals Oversteps Human Rights

Carol Grunewald

Animals rights and environmental activist Carol Grunewald works for the Humane Society of the United States in Washington, D.C. Formerly an editor with the magazine *The Animal Rights Agenda* and a Times Mirror newspaper reporter, Grunewald has written extensively on animal rights issues. In the following viewpoint, she decries the growing interest in the genetic engineering of animals to suit human purposes. This research, she says, will lead to further harm for animals and will endanger humans as well.

As you read, consider the following questions:

1. What two events does the author say were instrumental in spurring the growth of interest in animal genetic research?
2. According to Grunewald, in what ways are animals already worse off because of genetic engineering research?
3. What does Grunewald perceive as likely long-term consequences of continued research on animal genetic engineering?

It's probably no accident that some of the most fearsome monsters invented by the human mind have been composed of body parts of various animal—including human—species.

Ancient and mediaeval mythology teem with 'transgenic' creatures who have served through the ages as powerful symbols and movers of the human subconscious. In Greek mythology the Chimera—a hideous fire-breathing she-monster with the head of a lion, the body of a goat and a dragon's tail—was darkness incarnate and a symbol of the underworld.

At the beginning of the industrial or technological age, the collective consciousness conjured monsters from a new but related fear—the consequences of human interference with nature. Fears of science and technology gone out of control created the stories of *Dr. Jekyll and Mr. Hyde* and *Dr. Frankenstein.*

The contemporary monster is apt to be a real human being, but an amoral, sociopathic one—a Mengele or an Eichmann who imposes his evil will not in the heat of passion, but in cold detachment.

Deepest Human Fears

Our nightmares, our mythologies, our movies, our real-life monsters reveal many of our deepest human fears: of the unknown, of the unnatural, of science gone berserk and of the dark side of the human psyche. With such an intense subliminal heritage, no wonder many people are instinctively wary of the new and revolutionary science of genetic engineering—a science born just 15 years ago but which is already creating its own monsters. They have good reason to be afraid.

The goal of genetic engineering is to break the code of life and to re-form and 'improve' the biological world according to human specifications. It is the science of manipulating genes either within or between organisms. Genes are the fundamental and functional units of heredity; they are what make each of us similar to our species but individually different.

There are two astonishing aspects to this new science. For the first time, humankind has the capacity to effect changes in the genetic code of individual organisms which will be passed down to future generations.

Equally startling, humankind now has the ability to join not only various animal species that could never mate in nature but also to cross the fundamental biological barriers between plants and animals that have always existed.

Experiments have already produced a few animal monstrosities. 'Geeps', part goat, part sheep, have been engineered through the process of cell-fusion—mixing cells of goat and sheep embryos. A pig has been produced whose genetic structure was altered by the insertion of a human gene responsible for producing a growth hormone. The unfortunate animal (nick-named 'super-pig') is so riddled with arthritis she can barely stand, is nearly blind, and prone to developing ulcers and pneumonia. No doubt researchers will create many such debilitated and pain-racked animals until they get it right.

Custom-Designed Creatures

Meanwhile, the world's knowledge of genetic engineering is growing apace. Much of what is now only theoretically possible will almost certainly be realized. With the world's genetic pool at a scientist's disposal, the possibilities are endless. It's just a matter of time.

But two historic events spurred the growth in what is now referred to as the 'biotech industry'. In 1980 the US Supreme Court ruled, in a highly controversial 5-4 vote, that 'man-made' micro-organisms can be patented. Then in April 1987, without any public debate, the US Patent Officer suddenly announced that all forms of life—including animals but excluding human beings—may be considered 'human inventions'. These could qualify as 'patentable subject matter', provided they had been genetically engineered with characteristics not attainable through classical breeding techniques.

The economic incentives were impossible for researchers and corporations to resist. The genetic engineering of animals was a biological gold mine waiting to be exploited. In hope of getting rich off the 'inventions', scientists have so far 'created' thousands of animals nature could never have made. Now more than 90 patents are pending for transgenic animals, and some 7,000 are pending for genetically engineered plant and animal micro-organisms.

Until now animal rights activists have been the foremost opponents of genetic engineering. The reason: animals are already the worse for it. Because they are powerless, animals have always suffered at the hands of humankind. When a new technology comes along, new ways are devised to exploit them. But genetic engineering represents the most extreme and blatant form of animal exploitation yet.

Genetic engineers do not see animals as they are: inherently valuable, sentient creatures with sensibilities very similar to ours and lives of their own to live. To them, animals are mere biological resources, bits of genetic code that can be manipulated at will and 'improved' to serve human purposes. They can then be patented like a new toaster or tennis ball.

In a recent article, the US Department of Agriculture crows that '. . . the face of animal production in the twenty-first century could be . . . broilers blooming to market size 40 per cent quicker, miniature hens cranking out eggs in double time, a computer "cookbook" of recipes for custom-designed creatures'.

The trade journal of the American beef industry boasts that in the year 2014 farmers will be able to order 'from a Sears-type Catalog, specific breeds or mixtures of breeds of (genetically engineered) cattle identified by a model number and name. Just like the 2014's new model pick-up truck, new model animals can be ordered for specific purposes'.

A university scientist says, 'I believe it's completely feasible to specifically design an animal for a hamburger'.

A Canadian researcher speaking at a farmers' convention eagerly tells the group that 'at the Animal Research Institute we are trying to breed animals without legs and chickens without feathers'.

Huge profits are to be made from new cows, pigs, chickens and other farm animals whose genetic scripts will be written and 'improved' to grow faster and leaner on less food and on new foods such as sawdust, cardboard and industrial and human waste.

Genetic Engineering Harms Animals

Genetic engineering and other new biotechnologies, such as embryo transplantation, cloning and the creation of chimeras like the 'geep'—a combination of the genetic material of a sheep and a goat—are relatively recent developments. This means that, at present, there is a total lack of evidence that the welfare of animals subjected to these manipulations can be guaranteed, and that coincidental and contingent suffering to these animals will be avoided. It is wrong to presume or promise that as a result of the application of these new technologies the welfare of animals will not be placed in jeopardy, and that 'unnecessary' suffering will be avoided.

Michael Fox in *The Bio-Revolution: Cornucopia or Pandora's Box*, edited by Peter Wheale and Ruth McNally, 1990.

Researchers have been straining at the bit to design and patent new animal 'models' of human disease—living, breathing 'tools' who will be experimented to death in the laboratory. Scientists have also created 'medicine factories' out of mice by implanting in them human genes for producing human enzymes, proteins and drugs that can be harvested. Cows, sheep and other milk-producing animals have been targeted for further experimentation in this area.

Animals already suffer abominably in intensive-confinement factory farms and laboratories. Genetic manipulations will result in further subjugation of animals and increase and intensify their stress, pain and mental suffering.

But genetic engineering also imposes risks on wildlife and the environment. Many questions need to be asked. For example, what will happen when genetically-altered animals and plants are released into the environment? Once they're out there we can't get them back. What if they run amok? Carp and salmon are currently engineered to grow twice as large as they do in nature. But will they also consume twice as much food? Will they upset the ecological balance and drive other animal or plant species to extinction'?

Indeed, the genetic engineering of animals will almost certainly endanger species and reduce biological diversity. Once researchers develop what is considered to be the 'perfect carp' or 'perfect chicken' these will be the ones that are reproduced in large numbers. All other 'less desirable' species would fall by the wayside and decrease in number. The 'perfect' animals might even be cloned—reproduced as exact copies—reducing even further the pool of available genes on the planet.

Such fundamental human control over all nature would force us to view it differently. Which leads us to the most important examination of all: our values.

How Human?

'We need to ask ourselves what are the long term consequences for civilization of reducing all of life to engineering values'. These are the words of Foundation on Economic Trends President Jeremy Rifkin, the leading opponent of genetic engineering in the US. Rifkin warns that the effects of new technologies are pervasive. They reach far beyond the physical, deep into the human psyche and affect the well-being of all life on earth.

In the brave new world of genetic engineering will life be precious? If we could create living beings at will—and even replace a being with an exact clone if it died—would life be valued? The patenting of new forms of life has already destroyed the distinction between living things and inanimate objects. Will nature be just another form of private property?

The intermingling of genes from various species, including the human species, will challenge our view of what it means to be human. If we inject human genes into animals, for example, will they become part human? If animal genes are injected into humans will we become more animal? Will the distinctions be lost? And if so, what will the repercussions be for all life?

And will humans be able to create, patent, and thus own a being that is, by virtue of its genes, part human? In other words, how human would a creature have to be in order to be included in the system of rights and protections that are accorded to 'full humans' today?

We may already know the answer to that question. Chimpanzees share 99 per cent of our human genetic inheritance, yet nowhere in the world is there a law that prevents these nearly 100-per-cent human beings from being captured, placed in leg-irons, owned, locked in laboratory and zoo cages and dissected in experiments.

The blurring of the lines between humans and animals could have many interesting consequences. All of us (humans and animals) are really made of the same 'stuff' and our genes will be used interchangeably. Since we are already 'improving' animals to serve our needs, why not try and improve ourselves as well? With one small step, we could move from animal eugenics to human eugenics and, by means of genetic engineering, make the plans of the Nazis seem bumbling and inefficient.

Life as Property

Finally, who will control life? Genetic technology is already shoring up the mega-multinational corporations and consolidating and centralizing agribusiness. Corporate giants like General Electric, Du Pont, Upjohn, Ciba-Geigy, Monsanto, and Dow Chemical have multi-billion-dollar investments in genetic engineering technology. It is becoming increasingly clear that we are placing the well-being of the planet and all its inhabitants in the hands of a technological elite. Our scientists, corporations and military are playing with, and may eventually own, our genes.

The arrogance and foolishness of humankind! With everything on the planet existing just to be used and exploited—with nothing existing without a 'reason' and a 'use'—where is the joy of life? What is the reason for living?

People and animals are inseparable; our fates are inextricably linked. People are animals. What is good for animals is good for the environment is good for people. What is bad for them is bad for us.

The first line of resistance should be to scrap the patenting of animals. And the release of any genetically altered organisms into the environment should be prohibited.

Finally, we must remember that the mind that views animals as pieces of coded genetic information to be manipulated and exploited at will is the mind that would view human beings in a similar way. People who care about people should listen carefully to what Animals Rights activists and environmentalists have to say about obtaining justice for, and preserving the integrity of, *all* life.

Periodical Bibliography

The following articles have been selected to supplement the diverse views presented in this chapter.

Carol J. Adams   "Anima, Animus, Animal," *Ms.*, May/June 1991.

Christopher Anderson   "Monkey Business," *The New Republic*, November 16, 1992.

Animals' Agenda   Several articles on dissection in the classroom. November 1991.

Tom L. Beauchamp   "The Moral Standing of Animals in Medical Research," *Law, Medicine, & Health Care*, Spring/Summer 1992. Available from the American Society of Law & Medicine, 765 Commonwealth Ave., Boston, MA 02215.

Dennis L. Breo   "Animal Rights vs. Research? A Question of the Nation's Scientific Literacy," *JAMA*, November 21, 1990.

Richard Conniff   "Fuzzy-Wuzzy Thinking About Animal Rights," *Audubon*, November 1990.

David DeGrazia   "The Moral Status of Animals and Their Use in Research: A Philosophical Review," *Kennedy Institute of Ethics Journal*, March 1991. Available from Journals Publishing Division, Johns Hopkins University Press, 2715 N. Charles St., Baltimore, MD 21218-4319.

Kathleen Hart   "Making Mythical Monsters," *The Progressive*, March 1990.

Hastings Center Report   Special section, "Animals, Science, and Ethics," May/June 1990.

The Humanist   Several articles, July/August 1990.

Charles Marwick   "Additional Voices Heard in Support of Humane Animal Use in Research," *JAMA*, June 6, 1990.

Medical Ethics Advisor   "Transplant of Baboon Liver Raises Variety of Ethical Questions," September 1992. Available from American Health Consultants, Inc., 3525 Piedmont Rd. NE, Building Six, Suite 400, Atlanta, GA 30304.

The New Internationalist	Entire issue on biomedical ethics, January 1991.
Harriet Ritvo	"Toward a More Peaceable Kingdom," *Technology Review*, February/March 1992.
Stanley Schmidt	"Accept No Substitutes," *Analog Science Fiction & Fact*, June 1992. Available from Davis Publications, Inc., 380 Lexington Ave., New York, NY 10017.
Tom Stafford	"Animal Lib," *Christianity Today*, June 18, 1990.
Alice Steinbach	"Whose Life Is More Important: An Animal's or a Child's?" *Glamour*, January 1990.
Betsy Swart	"Innocent Casualties in the War on Drugs," *On the Issues*, Winter 1990. Available from CHOICES Women's Medical Center, Inc., 97-77 Queens Blvd., Forest Hills, NY 11374-3317.
Robert Wright	"Are Animals People Too?" *The New Republic*, March 12, 1990.

What Ethics Should Guide Genetic Research?

Biomedical Ethics

Chapter Preface

In 1865 Gregor Mendel, an Austrian botanist and monk, published a study of heredity in peas. This was the first published scientific work on genetics. Mendel's work eventually allowed scientists to develop an understanding of how all kinds of living things pass certain physical traits on to their offspring. In 1953 British biophysicist Francis Crick and American geneticist James Watson broke the human genetic code and built the first accurate model of DNA, the "building block" of human heredity. enabling further understanding of how people pass their traits on to their children. In 1988 scientists embarked on the Human Genome Project (HGP), an odyssey to completely map the human genome—that is, all the genetic material in a "typical" human chromosome. The project, moving more rapidly than its originally anticipated fifteen years, aims to catalogue three billion base pairs of nucleotides (subunits of the DNA molecule) before it is finished. Other scientists are simultaneously studying particular nucleotides or DNA "markers" in order to understand how they work and how they affect such things as human development, intelligence, and disease.

The HGP and its related genetic research have been surrounded by controversy from the beginning. Already scientists have discovered genetic knowledge that may enable them to cure or prevent cystic fibrosis, to predict susceptibility to certain types of cancer and other diseases, and to treat certain types of genetic abnormalities while a fetus is still in its mother's womb. They think they have also discovered genetic reasons for certain types of behavior and psychological traits.

Critics fear that the knowledge scientists are developing will be used not only to treat disease but also to engineer away traits that those in power consider abnormal or undesirable. The consequences, they believe, will be discrimination against anyone who does not fit the acceptable mold; possible unanticipated loss of desirable traits; and the growth of eugenics, the science of "breeding" people to improve the human race.

The authors in the following chapter debate the ethical course for genetic research and applications in the coming years.

> *"That DNA . . . does not constitute the 'essence'
> of human life, nor tell us 'what we are,' . . . are
> ideas that have become so strange that they are
> virtually unthinkable."*

Genetic Research Threatens the Concept of Humanness

Howard L. Kaye

The great advances in genetic knowledge over the past decade have alarmed many scientists and social commentators. In the following viewpoint, Howard L. Kaye, professor of sociology at Franklin and Marshall College in Lancaster, Pennsylvania, muses on the impact of genetic research on the human self-image. Kaye sees the danger that human beings could be viewed as little more than a collection of DNA molecules that can be altered at scientific will. He believes that if society allows this kind of attitude to become pervasive, humanity will lose its very essence. Kaye is the author of several books, including *The Social Meaning of Modern Biology*.

As you read, consider the following questions:

1. What does Kaye think is left out of definitions that explain humanity as a collection of malleable genetic characteristics?
2. What role does the author think the Human Genome Project is playing in dehumanizing society?
3. What objections does Kaye have to blindly accepting the idea that alcoholism, for example, may be eradicated biologically?

From Howard L. Kaye, "Are We the Sum of Our Genes?" *The Wilson Quarterly*, Spring 1992. Reprinted with permission.

Applause and a collective sigh of relief greeted the announcement in 1990 that a portion of the U.S. Human Genome Project's budget would be set aside each year for studies of the social and ethical implications of genetic research. Mindful of past experience with the atom and other revolutionary research put to uses that were not fully anticipated, scientists and administrators now seemed prepared to grapple with the possible uses and abuses of their work while it was underway.

Yet amid this celebration, the project's more profound implications are being overlooked. Many of the prominent scientists involved believe that the logical consequence of unlocking the gene's secrets will transcend science, requiring nothing less than a fundamental change in our understanding of human nature. With the mapping and sequencing of the human genome, they believe, will ultimately come knowledge of the genes associated with the whole range of human behavioral, mental, and moral traits. As these putative "genes for" such things as schizophrenia, alcoholism, homosexuality, manic-depression, intelligence, and criminality are "discovered" and publicized, the cumulative effect will be a transformation of how we understand ourselves: from moral beings, whose character and conduct is largely shaped by culture, social environment, and individual choice, to essentially biological beings, whose "fate," according to project head James Watson, "is in our genes."

This claim of Watson and other scientists is the latest episode in the controversial "return to biology" that began with the ethology of the 1960s and the sociobiology of the '70s and '80s. But whereas behavioral biologists during the past three decades, like the late-19th-century Social Darwinists before them, simply speculated about the possible hereditary bases and adaptive value of human traits and conduct, the geneticists of today believe they are poised to discover such genes and the biochemical pathways by which they shape our lives. To them, the Human Genome Project marks the culmination of more than a century of debate over the "implications" of modern biology that began with Darwin's *Origin of Species* (1859) and Francis Galton's *Hereditary Genius* (1869)—a debate lucidly chronicled in Carl Degler's recent *In Search of Human Nature*. . . .

Granting Too Much to Science

Whatever particular forms it has taken, the debate has always centered on the "implications" and "logical consequences" of the biological sciences for our understanding of human nature and culture. Today, however, faced by the prospect of an increased capacity and desire to intervene in the human genome, I believe that we must change the terms of the debate and give up this misguided quest. To think in terms of "implications" and "logical consequences" is to suggest that certain facts or propositions about human social behavior are so inseparably entwined with certain facts or propositions about biology that if the biological statement is true, the social statement follows necessarily.

"Implication" suggests a connection that is objective and logical. Yet is this really the case, or do we not thereby grant too much to science—ultimately the ability to tell us objectively who we are by nature—and too little to ourselves? Does any natural scientific proposition logically entail some significant human conclusion, or is this connection derived from other sources? Does relativity in physics, for example, "imply" moral relativity, as was argued earlier in this century? Does Darwinian theory "imply" the falseness of the biblical account of creation, as many have claimed for over a century? Does the proposition that an organism is "only DNA's way of making more DNA" imply that we and our culture are also "survival machines" built by natural selection to preserve and replicate our "immortal genes"? And finally, does the discovery of genetic correlates to the full range of human capacities and conduct truly imply the knowledge that "fate is in our genes"? . . .

The recognition that natural selection acting on the genome can affect behavioral characteristics has stimulated much valuable research. Nevertheless, to argue that the findings reveal "the essence of humanity," as Christopher Wills does, or the "objective criteria" by which human conduct must ultimately be judged, as political theorist Roger Masters does, and the proper means for making ourselves, in Watson's words, "a little better," is an interpretation of nature and of man that is more metaphysical than scientific. . . .

Unsatisfactory Guide to Human Nature

As our latest attempt at dropping some moral anchor, biology may prove as ambiguous and unsuccessful as previous scientific moralities—and perhaps even more harmful. Our current infatuation with biology, unlike that of a century ago, is occurring at a time when the humanities and social sciences have declared moral bankruptcy, thus depriving us of a vital part of the collective memory we need to regulate and resist our increased capacity for genetic manipulation. This sort of amnesia is painfully apparent, for example, in Wills's discussion of genetic influences on criminal behavior. Pointing to the common social backgrounds of police and criminals, Wills asks rhetorically, "Why should one group be law-abiding and the other not, if criminal behavior is engendered entirely by the environment?" For Wills, environmental and genetic determinism are apparently the only choices. What the former cannot explain must be attributed to the latter. Wedding a crude sociological determinism to an equally crude biology, Wills, like all for whom "nature and nurture" or "heredity and environment" are the only legitimate categories for understanding human life, utterly ignores the irreducible element of individual will, choice, and responsibility.

How are we to resist such irresponsible assertions—and the actions potentially sanctioned by them—if our scientists and opinion makers have forgotten what it means to be a moral and cultural being endowed, in Max Weber's words, "with the capacity and the will to take a deliberate attitude towards the world and to lend it significance"?

Playing God

Should biotechnology be allowed to play God? The implications are frightening. And alarm bells are being rung, not least by scientists themselves:

'We do not know what life is, and yet we manipulate it as if it were an inorganic salt solution,' says Dr Edwin Chagaff, Professor Emeritus of biochemistry at Columbia University Medical School. 'Science is now the craft of manipulation, modification, substitution and deflection of the forces of nature.'

And we are, he warns, heading toward 'human husbandry' in which embryos will be mass-produced for experimental purposes. 'What I see coming is a gigantic slaughterhouse, a molecular Auschwitz, in which valuable enzymes, hormones and so on will be extracted instead of gold teeth.'

Dick Russell, *The New Internationalist*, April 1988.

Fortunately, most nonacademics have not forgotten. Years ago, while literary and scientific intellectuals were extolling sociobiology's ethic of survival and "the morality of the gene," I overheard a doorman (married and the father of three) complain to a co-worker, "I'm not really living, just surviving." This is a sentiment I suspect we have all heard or experienced, but what was this man really saying? In distinguishing between *human* life and *biological* life was he not expressing the presence of a "self" or "soul" within him that aspired to a higher life, a more meaningful and fulfilling life than the life of biological survival and reproduction he was leading? Unlike our biologists, structural social scientists, and poststructural humanists, he recognized that we are meaning-craving and meaning-creating animals who aspire, however perversely, to the good. To understand such a nature, which desires "the good's being one's own always" and

256

which experiences the pain of shame, resentment, and guilt at our inadequacy, Plato's *Symposium* remains a better guide than E. O. Wilson's *Sociobiology*. It is not that Plato's biology is better than Wilson's but that the question of human nature is not simply a biological one, no matter how many genetic correlates of character are discovered. Our capacity for culture—understood not in the trivial biological sense as all nongenetic means that enable organisms to adapt to their environments, but in its properly human sense as that system of ideals, practices, and prohibitions that comes into being both to protect us from nature and from ourselves and "for the sake of living well"—may certainly be the product of natural selection. Our capacities for reason, symbolic expression, and imagination; our aspirations for esteem and respect; and our qualities of curiosity and self-consciousness all may have evolutionary origins and may have contributed to our species' biological success. But they have long since taken on applications and ends that transcend the narrowly biological and may at times contradict it. Indeed this need to dream of, reflect on, and feel shame before goods and ideals detached from and even contrary to both our "innate behavioral repertoire" and our ultimate biological ends is both our greatness and our curse. Nevertheless, it is precisely this capacity that is under attack, now on three fronts, as the natural sciences, social sciences, and humanities close in on their quarry: the self or soul.

Altering Our Self-Image

It is this attempt to redefine fundamentally how we conceive of ourselves as human beings, and thus how we conceive of a good and proper life, that makes contemporary biological naturalism so culturally radical in its potential consequences. Yet however inadequate and even harmful this perspective may be, however unfounded its claim to the status of "scientific implications" for its moral prescriptions, it has indeed begun to alter our self-conception. This is not because scientific knowledge has social *implications* but because it has had and will continue to have social *impact*. . . .

In the years to come, I expect this redefinition of ourselves as essentially biological beings to continue and to have even greater influence on individual actions and public policy. But whereas this once was the work of scientists addressing the public directly in works that were explicitly philosophical and manifestly seeking to convert, its continued development will, I fear, be far more indirect and insidious. The Human Genome Project will play a crucial role, but not simply through its discoveries in the laboratory. Instead, I expect that the cumulative effect of the ways such knowledge is likely to be interpreted for and by the broader public will push us, like sleepwalkers, toward the biologizing of our lives in both thought and practice.

Rethinking Free Will

I think what needs to be reexamined is what it means to talk about genes. We need to rethink what it means to talk about genetic determinism, equally for physiological traits and behavioral traits. If we accept the framework that human genetics provides us for all things physiological, we're not going to have a leg to stand on when it comes to behavioral traits. There's no question that the claims for behavioral genetics that will have any durability will be more complicated than the claims for most physiology. You're not going to be able to make credible claims for single gene determination of personality traits. But I don't have any doubt that they are going to be able to make credible claims for multi-gene "determination" of personality traits. . . .

The typical response of genetic determinists is to say: "People make a terrible mistake, they forget about free will. Just because genes determine our behavior doesn't mean we can't override our genes by the force of our free will."

Well, where do they think free will is going to come from? It's always possible, if you're committed liberal individuals, to bring in that specter of free will somewhere, but it makes less and less sense as molecular genetics proceeds. Especially as it proceeds into the domain of neurobiology, there's less and less room for this specter of free will.

Evelyn Keller Fox, *Socialist Review,* April/June 1991.

When a scientist such as Harvard's E. O. Wilson candidly acknowledges that the particular vision of human nature and culture he is advocating is drawn from the "mythology" of scientific materialism, the thoughtful reader is in a position to recognize Wilson's work for what it is—metaphysical speculation and natural theology—and evaluate it accordingly. Yet when the public reads in the newspaper of "genes for" various human attributes and behaviors and of the means for altering the human "blueprint" in seemingly desirable ways, few are able to recognize the moral and philosophical commitments that lie behind such statements. Yet such commitments are powerfully present, however unconscious or concealed behind "descriptive" language. When George Cahill of the Howard Hughes Medical Institute asserts that the Human Genome Project is "going to tell us everything. Evolution, disease, everything will be based on what's in that magnificent tape called DNA," the "everything" he means is everything worth knowing about life. When Maynard Olson of Washington University states that "genetics is the core science of biology and increasingly it's going to be the way that people think about life," he is not offering just a prediction but a moral prescription: Genetics is how we *ought* to think about life. When Robert Sinsheimer, the prominent scientist who helped launch the drive for a genome project in 1985, tells us that it will provide "the complete set of instructions for making a human being," he certainly ignores everything else that goes into the making of a human being. More ominous, however, is his emphasis on "making," for this is the same Robert Sinsheimer who in 1973 advocated the conscious direction of human evolution toward a "higher state" through eugenics as the only unifying goal left that could save us from our cultural despair.

Reductionist Quest

Heading the Human Genome Project is, of course, James Watson, codiscoverer of the structure of the DNA molecule. For Watson, the genome project is quite simply the culmination of his reductionist quest for understanding all of life including "ourselves at the molecular level." With this understanding we can and should increasingly control our fate. After all, why not? "A lot of people say they're worried about changing our genetic instructions," Watson acknowledges, "but those [instructions] are just a product of evolution designed to adapt us for certain conditions that may not exist today. . . . [So] why not make ourselves a little better suited for survival? . . . That's what I think we'll do. We'll make ourselves a little better."

The point here is not to raise the specter of mad scientists, hell-bent on eugenics, in charge of a multibillion-dollar government research project with important medical and political potential. Nor is it to suggest that a majority of researchers participating in the project share this metaphysical and social agenda. It is instead to argue that such pronouncements may have an important impact on public perception, public understanding, and ultimately public response to emerging biological knowledge and technologies. So pervasive is this highly reductive and deterministic view of life that it passes for self-evident and unproblematic scientific fact among those science writers and journalists who seek to keep the public informed about developments in biology. Newspapers and other media constantly refer to the genome as "the blueprint for a human being," "the formula for life" that "dictates . . . how an individual confronts the world" and that contains "the very essence" of our lives. They trumpet the discovery of "genes for" cancer, schizophrenia, manic-depression, and other maladies. In the *Philadelphia Inquirer* last fall, it was put quite simply: "Everything about us . . .

is determined by genes."

Even those critical of some developments in modern biology find it difficult to escape from its reductive language. Robert Wright of the *New Republic,* in a highly caustic piece on Watson and the genome project, nevertheless adheres to what Watson's colleague Francis Crick dubbed the "Central Dogma" of molecular biology: that DNA makes RNA, RNA makes protein, and "proteins (to oversimplify just a bit) are us." The "implications" of such a dogma appear clear. DNA, as shaped by natural selection and chance, essentially determines who we are and how we live, yet like any "blueprint" can be altered to fit new needs.

That human beings, and perhaps other organisms as well, are more than their DNA "blueprints" or the sum of their proteins; that DNA, however "magnificent" a tape it may be, does not constitute the "essence" of human life, nor tell us "what we are," in Watson's words, let alone who we are; that it is both incorrect and irresponsible to speak of having discovered "genes for alcoholism" or genes that "cause" schizophrenia, are ideas that have become so strange that they are virtually unthinkable. Yet because they have become unspoken and unthinkable, many will want to take actions and advocate policies on the basis of what passes for scientific fact.

Dehumanizing Misconceptions

When the news media announced the discovery of a "gene for alcoholism" in 1990, I recall mentioning to a colleague in chemistry that such language was dangerously misleading. After all, the research of Drs. Ernest Noble and Kenneth Blum had only suggested a possible genetic component contributing indirectly to the alcoholism of *some* individuals. To speak of a "gene for alcoholism" both exaggerates the degree of genetic influence and seems to attribute all forms and cases of alcoholism to the same biological cause. The study, moreover, has yet to be replicated by others and involved research on only 70 brains. Much to my surprise, the chemist strongly disagreed: "Now wait a minute! This may be a very important piece of knowledge," he said, "for it might mean that the best way of treating the problem of alcoholism is through its biological causes."

He was hardly alone in making the jump to possible biological interventions. Noble and Blum plan to develop a blood test within five years that would detect the presence of the relevant dopamine receptor gene so that screening and treatment by drugs can begin. Forgetting for a moment that the gene identified seems to be correlated with something vaguely defined as "pleasure-seeking activity" in general and not simply some cases of alcoholism, and ignoring temporarily the potentially devastating, stigmatizing effects of such screening, there is still a shocking lack of awareness that the question of the "best way" to treat a problem such as alcoholism is not purely a question of efficiency, speed, or cost. It is a moral and political question as well, or at least it is if we recognize that we are dealing both with a problem that has important social, cultural, and psychological causes and with a being who possesses a potentially free and responsible soul that ought to be respected. It may even be possible that the "best way" morally to treat such a person may not be the most cost-effective way.

In the years to come cases like this will only proliferate. Regular "scientific breakthroughs" will torment and excite us, yielding genetic "determinants" for dozens of traits and attributes, both desirable and undesirable. Powerful economic and political interests, coupled with the understandable desire of individual human beings to maximize the well-being of themselves and their children, will continue to tempt us to pursue courses of biological intervention that will dehumanize us all, unwittingly, in the name of scientific progress, individual freedom, and compassion. Yet the road to such dehumanization in action begins with our prior dehumanization in thought—our forgetting the kind of beings we are and our construction of a new self-definition seemingly sanctioned by the biological sciences which, in their ignorance and ambition, encourage us to forget.

"The emerging knowledge of genetic causation of morally deplorable behavior is an enlarging factor in the search to understand personal and moral therapy of the whole . . . person. "

Genetic Research Broadens the Understanding of Humanness

J. Robert Nelson

Many people who hold strong religious beliefs are uneasy with the conclusions of modern science regarding human nature. They often view science as an affront challenging the tenets of free will and God-based creation. J. Robert Nelson, however, sees science as providing information to stimulate fuller understanding of humanity and its place in creation. Director of the Institute of Religion at Texas Medical Center in Houston, and a member of the United Methodist Genetic Science Task Force, Nelson urges people to keep an open mind to science and to seek ways scientific knowledge can be applied to improve the human condition.

As you read, consider the following questions:

1. What impact does Nelson think the Human Genome Project will have on the understanding of what it means to be human?
2. According to Nelson, what distinguishes the materialistic view of life from the spiritual or idealistic view?
3. What are some of the positive things the author thinks genetic research can contribute to human knowledge?

From J. Robert Nelson, "What Is Life?" *Christian Social Action*, January 1991. Reprinted with permission.

One series of questions put to Christians by the Human Genome Initiative (a joint project of the US Department of Energy and the National Institutes of Health) is this: do the emerging data of genetic science require a reassessment of some traditional theological concepts of human life, human behavior and moral responsibility? Would such changes of theoretical and theological concepts merely indicate a more sophisticated scientific knowledge on the part of religious thinkers about the constantly immutable human organism? Or is a changing concept needed to account for a changing, evolving phenomenon called human life?

People who adhere to a religious faith that teaches a static view of nature and a pessimistic view of human history are not disposed to expect beneficial results from the modern life sciences. Their stance is defensive against the findings, in particular, of the paleontology and developmental biology of the human species. Data that suggest an evolving change of humans from primordial aeons to the present and beyond are dangerous to their religious doctrine. . . .

The Christian religious faith, which has actually facilitated the rise of modern experimental science, also enables persons to be tolerant of change and hopeful for the future. Here there is no weakening or diluting the belief in God as primordial Creator and continuing Sustainer of the cosmos. Neither is there surrender of conviction that humanity is uniquely God-related and primary among all other organic creatures. These beliefs make room for evolving modifications of human life, whether by natural or humanly contrived causes. And they generate an expectant, positive anticipation of progress in improving both individual and social life through the contributions of fruitful research and judiciously employed technology.

Sudden change cannot be easily assimilated, however; not even by persons who are open and friendly toward science. In the field of molecular biology, new knowledge keeps bubbling up to be reported in journals and popular media. It bubbles not like cool water in spring, but like liquid boiling furiously in a geyser.

The molecular geneticists have already opened a large window, so to speak, on the microscopic double helix of paired nucleotides (basic structural units of RNA [ribonucleic acid, associated with the control of cellular chemical activities] and DNA [deoxyribonucleic, the molecular basis of heredity in many organisms]) that constitute the DNA molecule. Now they are planning to expose a vast panorama of the estimated 100,000 genes in each human cell.

Gene Mapping

Speaking in Boston at the 1988 meeting of the American Association for the Advancement of Science, Dr. Victor A. McCusick of the Johns Hopkins University made a trenchant remark about the effect of the gene-mapping project. He said that from the time of Vesalius of Padua until now—400 years—we have known human physiology only by empirical description. Now we can have a physiological knowledge consisting of genetic information: no longer only the body's physical characteristics and chemistry, but its cellular constituency and genetic potential. Just as the marvelous new electronic scanning and magnetic resonance imaging machines give us an inside view of parts of the body, the gene mapping and sequencing will afford a look inside the cells and inside the chromosomes (where genes reside).

Genes Show Humans Are Connected to All Life

Not only do we look upon the human race as having tremendous variation; we look upon ourselves as having an infinite potential. To recognize that we are determined, in a certain sense, by a finite collection of information that is knowable will change our view of ourselves. It is the closing of an intellectual frontier, with which we will have to come to terms. . . .

One consequence of the human genome project is that we will see more and more clearly how connected all life really is. Research in early development tells us that the genes that form our bodies are similar to the genes that produce worms and fruit flies and every complicated organism. Those genes were created before the branching off of any of the higher organisms that are on the earth today. The data base of the human genome, coupled with our knowledge of the genetic makeup of model organisms, promises to reveal patterns of genes and to show us how we ourselves are embedded in the sweep of evolution that created our world.

Walter Gilbert, *The Code of Codes*, 1992.

When we speak of chromosomes, genes and nucleotides, we must use inadequate adjectives: small, tiny, microscopic; 20 angstroms in diameter, equaling 79 billionths of an inch; infinitesimal! A molecule of human DNA can be seen by electronic microscope, enlarged thousands of times. We know it is like a pair of double twisted strings, joined by pairs of nucleic acids at 3 billion points. The molecule is too small to be seen without an electron microscope. And yet, if those chains of genes were drawn out of their tight packing in one molecule, they would be seen to be almost a meter in length.

It is almost impossible to visualize one of the 100,000 genes on that chain; it is still difficult to conceptualize the inherent power of those genes to determine what kinds of organic cellular life they will produce. We describe them in popular parlance as "building blocks" of life, or "blueprints" of organisms; as being "programmed" or "wired" to produce protein for any one of the countless differing parts of the body. But those metaphors illustrate the gene's purposes very poorly and explain their activity not at all. Building blocks are crude and lifeless. Blueprints are just the expression of the architect's intelligence and imagination; they can achieve nothing by themselves. And the computer analogy of programming presupposes a person who invents the software and a machine to let it function.

It is no wonder that the unfolding mystery of the gene is stimulating a new era of philosophical and theological thinking about the nature of organic life in general and of human life in particular. The question humans have asked wistfully for as long as there has been self-conscious reflection is, "What is life?"

Concepts of Life

In general, two kinds of theories are offered to answer that question. We call one "materialistic"; we call the other "spiritual" or "idealistic."

The materialistic concept of life was advanced in ancient philosophy by Democritus among the Greeks and by Lucretius among the Romans. They believed that all organic systems and the power of living consisted essentially of hard, material atoms. They invented the word a-tom to say that it was irreducible; it could not be cut any finer. The spiritual idea of life arose even earlier in India, in the obscure origins of Hinduism. It was given maximum and enduring currency in the West by Plato and a long succession of philosophers called Neoplatonists. The core of this view is the belief that the essence of life is the soul, the spirit, or the mind. These are eternal. The physical manifestations of the body are only transitory appearances.

To the present day, biological research and philosophical biology have been pursued within the contrary tension of these two notions of life. The history of that tension and of the arguments to overcome the contradiction is a red thread of continuity in the history of all science. And the implications for philosophy, religion, theology and ethics cannot be separated from that history. Research in molecular biology and biochemistry is rapidly discovering heretofore unknown and surprising characteristics of the DNA molecule as the quintessential unit of life. And the new knowledge apparently gives support and comfort to both the materialists and the idealists, while equally preventing either one of them from claiming to have the true concept of life. Let me explain.

No one can reasonably disagree with the explanation of the structure and activity of the DNA molecule as the interaction of chemicals. Just as our entire written language is based upon the alphabet—A,B,C to Z—we know that the units of living matter have a four-lettered alphabet; A for adenine, G for guanine, T for thymine and C for cytosine. Combined with a sugar and a phosphate group, these compositions of atoms of carbon, hydrogen, nitrogen and oxygen produce the 20 amino acids, which in turn are the elements of proteins.

The Source of Energy

Deeper than the chemical structure of cells and genes is the emerging knowledge of atomic physicists about the very source of energy. So it would seem that the materialistic, or mechanistic, concept of life has been given a double warrant by the molecular biologists and the nuclear physicists. It all reduces down to physical-chemical energy. Whatever happens at the atomic and molecular level is simply due to random chance. There is no plan or purpose in nature. In this reductionist's view of life, all biogenesis, mutation, evolutionary development, morphology (a branch of biology dealing with form and structure of animals), health or disease, sensibility, behavior, mental activity—everything reduces by descending levels to the elementary electrical energy of the atom, be it a wave or a particle.

And yet—the "and yet" is extremely important—the very physical theory of energy being worked out today gives strength to the argument that energy and matter are themselves the expressions of an inexplicable force. We hesitate to call it a spiritual power or a metaphysical reality. And we must be careful, whatever our faith and piety might be, to invoke too readily the name of God or presence of divinity, while still leaving open the possibility of that invocation.

The new genetic science gives the same signals to both the mechanistic materialists and the absolute idealists, or spiritualists: namely, there is probably truth in the intuition that human life is an inseparable admixture of material and spiritual dimensions. They constitute a unity in the human being that we have come to express in medical terminology by a single adjective: "psychosomatic." "Psychosomatic" means the unity of soul and body, of spirit and matter, in the whole person. Used as a medical term, it is rather new. But its meaning is ancient, going back mainly to the Bible, and to the Hebraic insight set forth in the Old Testament and developed in the New Testament.

Based upon this biblical anthropology, an accepted model of the human person has prevailed in Western civilization. It is still considered to be normal and normative by a probable majority of people of this heritage. According to this view, a generic human, man or woman, consists of the physical body, in the head of which is a brain of large size and almost limitless capabilities.

The brain is the locus of the mind; but somehow the mind transcends the physico-chemical activity of the brain and the neurosensory system of the body. This transcendence is palpably demonstrated by the voluntary exercise of the will in making decisions and directing the actions of the body. The relation of the brain to mind is thus described by some as interaction. New research in endocrinology of the brain as well as in psychic phenomena seems to strengthen the notion of mind-brain interaction. Beyond both, however, in this common view, is the unique soul of each individual person, wherein the deepest attributes of selfhood are to be found. The soul is also believed to be the living link to metaphysical reality and intelligent power. In personal and theistic terms, this reality is called "God."

Genetic Determinism

Such an understanding of human life is just as widely held today as it was before 1953. It has been challenged mainly by psychologists of the behaviorist school who rejected the belief in human free will. After 1953, this belief is more strongly challenged and rejected for reason of genetic determination. The total rejection need not be accepted; but the challenge of DNA is serious and inescapable. It must be met. It is the challenge of genetic determinism.

Potential Beyond Status Quo

Human beings—indeed all currently existing species—are highly evolved, extraordinarily complex, and marvelously well adapted to their natural ecology. We should be very wary indeed about altering components of this system until we have a good understanding of what role the components play in the overall organization of the system. However, it is one thing to suggest we act cautiously, keeping in mind that there are generally good evolutionary reasons for an organism's genome being the way it is. It is quite another thing to suppose natural selection cannot be improved on. To accept that view is to accept the Panglossian assumption that the status quo is the best of all possible worlds. And that assumption is simply not true.

Stephen P. Stich, *Values and Public Policy*, 1992.

In what ways are you and I determined by our genomes, which we inherit almost entirely from our parents and forebears? I say "almost" entirely because of a relatively small number of genetic changes, or mutations, that take place in our bodies during our development before birth. These may be caused by infections, chemical toxins, alcohol, x-rays, drugs and diseases of the mother-to-be.

We think first of basic physical characteristics: skin and hair color, facial structure, eyes, stature and general appearance. Then come secondly, genetic diseases, nearly 4,000 of which have now been identified. Many of them can be predicted on the simple basis of familial genetic histories or by the more sophisticated methods of linkage analysis, gene probes and markers, called Restriction Fragment Length Polymorphisms.

Prenatal analysis of maternal and fetal tissue is rapidly expanding to confirm or refute genetic predictions and to discover abnormalities that could not have been predicted. The list of these discoverable and predictable diseases keeps growing as researchers succeed in finding their deleterious genes: cystic fibrosis, Duchenne muscular dystrophy, dwarfism, Huntington's disease, polycystic kidney disease, sickle cell anemia, retinoblastoma, alpha-antitrypsin deficiency, PKU (phenylketonuria), Lesch-Nyhan disease, the hemophilias and neural tube defects such as spina bifida.

Susceptibilities

Third, beyond the manifest diseases as such, are the susceptibilities to certain diseases. The famous oncogenes (related to tumor formations) give clear indications of vulnerability to 50 various cancers. Other tests show dispositions to heart disease, arthritis, diabetes, as well as the neural and mental disorders, manic depression, schizophrenia. Unlike the clearly defined genetic diseases that are heritable, and that usually manifest themselves during fetal and newborn stages of life, these susceptibilities can be predicted to appear eventually toward the middle or end of life.

Fourth are the predictable dispositions toward various kinds of abnormal behavior. These are not diseases in the strict sense, but pre-determined patterns of personal behavior. Some are of a psychopathic nature, such as schizophrenia and manic depression. They are not morally reprehensible, as though due to deliberate choice; yet they are on the border of behavior for which our society tends to hold people responsible. But there are other types of behavior morally decried by the arbiters of a good society, but toward which the person may be genetically disposed; or more strongly, these may be genetically determined. Alcoholism is one of these; sexual aberration is another. Some researchers suggest that kleptomania (compulsive stealing) may have genetic causation. And even gambling may be caused. Compulsive inclination toward violent and criminal activity—the notorious XYY genotype—has recently been debated by geneticists and moralists. Controlled studies of identical twins, reared in differing environments but behaving in identical ways, give credibility to these theories, if not yet certainty.

The challenge that confronts us when we consider what is normal and morally correct about humanity becomes ever clearer. To what extent are the pathologies of personal behavior due to free choice? To what extent due to our genomes? Does objectionable behavior belong to the same categories as abnormal physical structure, congenital diseases and susceptibilities to disease? Or, to turn the question from negative to positive values: is good behavior something to be learned only by environmental and cultural influence and practiced as a matter of mature will and free choice? Or is goodness, such as altruistic behavior observed in humans or termites, so genetically determined as to ensure the survival of the species? As the sociobiologists have expressed it, the only purpose of genes is to reproduce more of the same, whatever the organism may be.

In a sense, sociobiologists have simply carried to extreme lengths the theory of genetic influence on behavior that is widely accepted in respect to physical characteristics and diseases. From the observed behavior of social insects, birds and mammals, they have extrapolated the principles of determination and applied it to humankind. Of course, like all others who study biology, they have to take account of the influences of environmental factors on growth, health and behavior.

To reject this extreme ideology, with all of its inhumane implications, does not make us blind to the demonstrated truth about the range of genetic effects on human behavior. Just as rapidly expanding knowledge of the genes that cause diseases is driving researchers to devise methods of gene therapy, so also the emerging knowledge of genetic causation of morally deplorable behavior is an enlarging factor in the search to understand personal and moral therapy of the whole, psychosomatic person. The task is as mandatory as it is awesome.

> *"People have a right to make what they want of their lives. . . . Minimal constraint is as good a principle in genetic law as in any other."*

Genetic Engineering Should Be Unrestricted

The Economist

The new genetic knowledge offers the possibility of humans being able to design their own evolution—both individually and societally. While many people find this alarming, the following viewpoint asserts that it is an exciting and promising opportunity that should not be avoided. The viewpoint, an editorial in the *Economist*, a London newspaper, argues that people should have as much choice as possible in determining what their lives will be like.

As you read, consider the following questions:

1. Does the author seem to agree with Sigmund Freud's statement that "biology is destiny"? How does the author interpret this statement?
2. The author implies that changes brought about by genetics are comparable to those brought about by drugs or surgery. Do you think the comparison is valid? Explain.
3. According to the author, why will "biology . . . be best when it is a matter of choice"?

"Biology is destiny." Though the years have been unkind to Sigmund Freud's thought, that notion sounds fresher now than when he said it. In the 1950s the threads of destiny were given form when Francis Crick and James Watson elucidated the double-helix structure of DNA. In the 1960s the language of genes, in which the messages stored on DNA are written, was translated; biology, and much else, began to change. Genes are blamed for everything from cancer to alcoholism. People worry about being made ineligible for jobs because of disease susceptibilities they never knew they had; fetuses are aborted because of faults in their genes; criminals are defined by the bar-codes of their genetic fingerprints.

Gene Therapy

At first glance, genetic therapy—the nascent art of giving sick people new genes to alleviate their illness—looks like the apotheosis of this trend towards reducing human life to a few short sequences of DNA. But although its advent means people will be talking in the language of genes even more than they already do, the way they talk will change. They will not be passively reading out the immutable genetic lore passed down from generation to generation. They will not be receiving orders; they will be giving them. The birth of genetic therapy marks the beginning of an age in which man has the power to take control of his genes and make of them what he will.

At the moment, gene therapy is a small field on the fringes of medicine and biotechnology. Genes carry descriptions of proteins, the molecules that do most of the body's work; if someone is missing a gene, they will be missing a protein, and may thus suffer a deficiency or disease. If a gene or set of genes runs amok, cancer can result. The gene-therapists aim to provide the body with genes to make good its deficiencies and problems. If their field had grown as fast as the stacks of ethical reports and regulatory procedures that surround it, it would already be big business. As it is, after years of discussion, it is only now starting to blossom. Therapies are being tried on people around the world (though in tiny numbers) and new ways of delivering genes are being devised. A torrent of raw material for tomorrow's therapies is flowing from the human genome programme, which plans to have a description of every gene and every scrap of DNA found in the body by the early years of the next century.

Many hear echoes of eugenics at every mention of the gene, and look at this progress with fear. Present research, though, provides no cause for alarm, just an occasion for the routine caution with which all medical advances must be treated. From one point of view, gene therapies are transplants; from another, they are just drug treatments with the added twist that the drug

271

is being made inside the body. There already exist sets of rules for trying out drugs. The question of the drug's provenance is of secondary importance, as long as its manufacture can be shown to be safe. Experimental gene therapy has satisfied regulators on that count, so far.

"So far," though, is only the beginning. Beyond today's gene therapy, which is a specialised form of medicine not that dissimilar to others, lie far more controversial possibilities: changing genes for non-medical reasons, and changing genes wholesale in such a way that the new genes are passed on from generation to generation. At present, therapists aim at genes that are clearly villains, and the therapies last at most as long as the patient, and often only as long as a transient set of cells. But what of genes that might make a good body better, rather than make a bad one good? Should people be able to retrofit themselves with extra neurotransmitters, to enhance various mental powers? Or to change the colour of their skin? Or to help them run faster, or lift heavier weights?

Humans Make Choices

While the dilemmas of genetic research give many reasons to pause and reflect, they do not justify slowing or stopping the research itself. In many cases, the best way to eliminate dilemmas—and protect human life—is to push back genetic frontiers. Admittedly, there are risks involved. The more we master genes, the more options—many of them morally questionable—we will have. But making choices, after all, is what being human is all about.

Joel L. Swerdlow, *Wilson Quarterly*, Spring 1992.

Yes, they should. Within some limits, people have a right to make what they want of their lives. The limits should disallow alterations clearly likely to cause harm to others. Even if the technology allowed it, people should not be allowed to become psychopaths at will, or to alter their metabolism so that they are permanently enraged. Deciding which alterations sit in this forbidden category would have to be done case by case, and in some cases the toss may be passionately argued. But so it is with all constraints on freedom. Minimal constraint is as good a principle in genetic law as in any other.

People may make unwise choices. Though that could cause them grief, it will be remediable. That which can be done, can be undone; people need no more be slaves to genes they have chosen than to genes they were born with. To keep that element of choice, however, one thing must be out of bounds. No one should have his genes changed without his informed consent; to force genetic change on another without his consent is a violation of his person, a crime as severe as rape or grievous bodily harm. There may be subtle social pressures to choose certain traits; but there is often social pressure for all sorts of things, and it does not deny the subject free will.

God and Nature

Some will object, in the names of God and nature. Religious beliefs may strongly influence people's decisions about what, if any, engineering they undergo. They should not be allowed to limit the freedoms of unbelievers. In that it uses natural processes for human ends, gene therapy is as natural, or as unnatural, as most medicine. But even the artificial carries no moral stigma. The limits imposed by nature are practical, not moral. The body does not have infinite capacities—gains in one ability usually mean losses in others. Natural selection always seeks to fit the balance of abilities to a given environment, and abilities it has optimised may prove hard to enhance. Substantial improvements in human intellect, for example, may not be possible using genes alone.

All this refers to the engineering of cells in the bulk of the body, "somatic" cells which pass no genes to the next generation. But to influence the early development of embryos, or to create radically different types of persons, requires a different approach, one that puts new genes into all cells—including the eggs and sperm, whence they can launch themselves into the next generation. This sort of "germ-line" therapy, with its long-term effects, brings to mind spectres of master races and *Untermenschen* that limited cell therapy does not.

One response to these worries, used by many scientists in the field, is to say that germ-line therapy is not an option. Prospective patients may disagree. Some conditions, which do their nasty work on small embryos, may for all practical purposes be treatable only by using germ-line therapy. As yet, no therapy for such conditions has been devised. If it is, it would not necessarily be ruled out; but it would be right to regulate it far more closely than regular, somatic-cell therapy. Germ-line therapy would be similar to major surgery on an unborn child incapable of informed consent. In such cases, it is commonly accepted that the parents are justified in acting in the child's interests. If they can show they are undeniably doing so, there similarly seems no ground for denying the gene therapy. But that undeniable interest will have to be the avoidance of a clear blight that would prevent the child, if not treated, from ever being able to take a similar decision about its future.

If somatic-cell therapy becomes common, if biological understanding becomes far more profound and if people show an abiding interest in transforming themselves, then a less conservative approach may prevail—not least because people would know that a child with genes foisted on it by its parents might be able to change them itself, come the time. In such a world, changing children may look less worrying; or it may look unnecessary. Not all change is genetic. Surgery can transform people too, as many transsexuals will testify; increasing intelligence may be easier with prosthetic computers than with rewired brains. The proper goal is to allow people as much choice as possible about what they do. To this end, making genes instruments of such freedom, rather than limits upon it, is a great step forward. With apologies to Freud, biology will be best when it is a matter of choice.

Genetic Engineering Should Be Restricted to Medical Therapy

W. French Anderson

Human genetic science is used almost exclusively today in a therapeutic manner. That is, it is used to diagnose and predict disease and other abnormalities, and it is being used, to a small extent, to alter abnormal or disease-carrying genes. In plant and animal science, however, geneticists have dramatically altered existing life-forms and created new ones. These latter accomplishments alarm many people, including the author of the following viewpoint, W. French Anderson, chief of the Laboratory of Molecular Hematology of the National Heart, Lung, and Blood Institute at the National Institutes of Health in Bethesda, Maryland. Anderson believes that altering human genes in any but a therapeutic way is both dangerous and unethical.

As you read, consider the following questions:

1. What are some examples of genetic manipulation that the author approves of?
2. How does Anderson distinguish between ethical and unethical uses of genetic knowledge?
3. List three of the major questions Anderson says are raised by genetic engineering for enhancement purposes.

From W. French Anderson, "Genetics and Human Malleability," *Hastings Center Report*, January/February 1990. Reprinted with permission.

Just how much can, and should we change human nature . . . by genetic engineering? Our response to that hinges on the answers to three further questions: (1) What *can* we do now? Or more precisely, what *are* we doing now in the area of human genetic engineering? (2) What *will* we be able to do? In other words, what technical advances are we likely to achieve over the next five to ten years? (3) What *should* we do? I will argue that a line can be drawn and should be drawn to use gene transfer only for the treatment of serious disease, and not for any other purpose. Gene transfer should never be undertaken in an attempt to enhance or "improve" human beings. . . .

It is clear that there are several applications for gene transfer that probably will be carried out over the next five to ten years. Many genetic diseases that are caused by a defect in a single gene should be treatable, such as ADA deficiency (a severe immune deficiency disease of children), sickle cell anemia, hemophilia, and Gaucher disease. Some types of cancer, viral diseases such as AIDS, and some forms of cardiovascular disease are targets for treatment by gene therapy. In addition, germline gene therapy, that is, the insertion of a gene into the reproductive cells of a patient, will probably be technically possible in the foreseeable future. . . .

But successful somatic cell gene therapy also opens the door for enhancement genetic engineering, that is, for supplying a specific characteristic that individuals might want for themselves (somatic cell engineering) or their children (germline engineering) which would not involve the treatment of a disease. The most obvious example at the moment would be the insertion of a growth hormone gene into a normal child in the hope that this would make the child grow larger. Should parents be allowed to choose (if the science should ever make it possible) whatever useful characteristics they wish for their children?

No Enhancement Engineering

A line can and should be drawn between somatic cell gene therapy and enhancement genetic engineering. Our society has repeatedly demonstrated that it can draw a line in biomedical research when necessary. The [1978] Belmont Report [a government-sponsored study on the protection of human research subjects] illustrates how guidelines were formulated to delineate ethical from unethical clinical research and to distinguish clinical research from clinical practice. Our responsibility is to determine how and where to draw lines with respect to genetic engineering.

Somatic cell gene therapy for the treatment of severe disease is considered ethical because it can be supported by the fundamental moral principle of beneficence: It would relieve human suffering. Gene therapy would be, therefore, a moral good. Under what circumstances would human genetic engineering not be a moral good? In the broadest sense, when it detracts from, rather than contributes to, the dignity of man. Whether viewed from a theological perspective or a secular humanist one, the justification for drawing a line is founded on the argument that, beyond the line, human values that our society considers important for the dignity of man would be significantly threatened.

Somatic cell enhancement engineering would threaten important human values in two ways: It could be medically hazardous, in that the risks could exceed the potential benefits and the procedure therefore cause harm. And it would be morally precarious, in that it would require moral decisions our society is not now prepared to make, and it could lead to an increase in inequality and discriminatory practices.

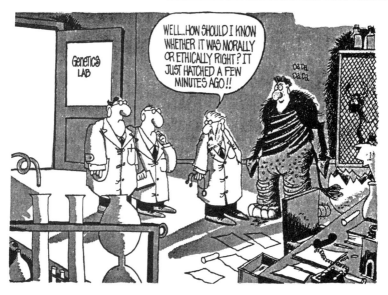

Ed Gamble for the *Florida Times Union*. Reprinted with permission.

Medicine is a very inexact science. We understand roughly how a simple gene works and that there are many thousands of housekeeping genes, that is, genes that do the job of running a cell. We predict that there are genes which make regulatory messages that are involved in the overall control and regulation of the many housekeeping genes. Yet we have only limited understanding of how a body organ develops into the size and shape it does. We know many things about how the central nervous system works—for example, we are beginning to comprehend how molecules are involved in electric circuits, in memory storage, in transmission of signals. But we are a long way from understanding thought and consciousness. And we are even further from understanding the spiritual side of our existence.

Even though we do not understand how a thinking, loving, interacting organism can be derived from its molecules, we are approaching the time when we can change some of those molecules. Might there be genes that influence the brain's organization or structure or metabolism or circuitry in some way so as to allow abstract thinking, contemplation of good and evil, fear of death, awe of a "God"? What if in our innocent attempts to improve our genetic make-up we alter one or more of those genes? Could we test for the alteration? Certainly not at present. If we caused a problem that would affect the individual or his or her offspring, could we repair the damage? Certainly not at present. Every parent who has several children knows that some babies accept and give more affection than others, in the same environment. Do genes control this? What if these genes were accidentally altered? How would we even know if such a gene were altered?

Tinkering with the Unknown

My concern is that, at this point in the development of our culture's scientific expertise, we might be like the young boy who loves to take things apart. He is bright enough to disassemble a watch, and maybe even bright enough to get it back together again so that it works. But what if he tries to "improve" it? Maybe put on bigger hands so that the time can be read more easily. But if the hands are too heavy for the mechanism, the watch will run slowly, erratically, or not at all. The boy can understand what is visible, but he cannot comprehend the precise engineering calculations that determined exactly how strong each spring should be, why the gears interact in the ways that they do, etc. Attempts on his part to improve the watch will probably only harm it. We are now able to provide a new gene so that a property involved in a human life would be changed, for example, a growth hormone gene. If we were to do so simply because we could, I fear we would be like that young boy who changed the watch's hands. We, too, do not really understand what makes the object we are tinkering with tick. . . .

Yet even aside from the medical risks, somatic cell enhancement engineering should not be performed because it would be morally precarious. Let us assume that there were no medical risks at all from somatic cell enhancement engineering. There would still be reasons for objecting to this procedure. To illustrate, let us consider some examples. What if a human gene were cloned that could produce a brain chemical resulting in markedly increased memory capacity in monkeys after gene transfer? Should a person be allowed to receive such a gene on request? Should a pubescent adolescent whose parents are both five feet tall be provided with a growth hormone gene on request? Should a worker who is continually exposed to an industrial toxin receive a gene to give him resistance on his, or his employer's request?

Three Problems

These scenarios suggest three problems that would be difficult to resolve: What genes should be provided; who should receive a gene; and, how to prevent discrimination against individuals who do or do not receive a gene.

We allow that it would be ethically appropriate to use somatic cell gene therapy for treatment of serious disease. But what distinguishes a serious disease from a "minor" disease from cultural "discomfort"? What is suffering? What is significant suffering? Does the absence of growth hormone that results in a growth limitation to two feet in height represent a genetic disease? What about a limitation to a height of four feet, to five feet? Each observer might draw the lines between serious disease, minor disease, and genetic variation differently. But all can agree that there are extreme cases that produce significant suffering and premature death. Here then is where an initial line should be drawn for determining what genes should be provided: treatment of serious disease.

If the position is established that only patients suffering from serious diseases are candidates for gene insertion, then the issues of patient selection are no different than in other medical situations: the determination is based on medical need within a supply and demand framework. But if the use of gene transfer extends to allow a normal individual to acquire, for example, a memory-enhancing gene, profound problems would result. On what basis is the decision made to allow one individual to receive the gene but not another: Should it go to those best able to benefit society (the smartest already?) To those most in need (those with low intelligence? But how low? Will enhancing memory help a mentally retarded child?)? To those chosen by a lottery? To those who can afford to pay? As long as our society lacks a significant consensus about these answers, the best way to make equitable decisions in this case should be to base them on the seriousness of the objective medical need, rather than on the personal wishes or resources of an individual.

Discrimination can occur in many forms. If individuals are carriers of a disease (for example, sickle cell anemia), would they be pressured to be treated? Would they have difficulty in

279

obtaining health insurance unless they agreed to be treated? These are ethical issues raised also by genetic screening and by the Human Genome Project. But the concerns would become even more troublesome if there were the possibility for "correction" by the use of human genetic engineering.

Finally, we must face the issue of eugenics, the attempt to make hereditary "improvements." The abuse of power that societies have historically demonstrated in the pursuit of eugenic goals is well documented. Might we slide into a new age of eugenic thinking by starting with small "improvements"? It would be difficult, if not impossible, to determine where to draw a line once enhancement engineering had begun. Therefore, gene transfer should be used only for the treatment of serious disease and not for putative improvements.

Our society is comfortable with the use of genetic engineering to treat individuals with serious disease. On medical and ethical grounds we should draw a line excluding any form of enhancement engineering. We should not step over the line that delineates treatment from enhancement.

"The incomparable relief I felt at finally being free of . . . uncertainty [is] a feeling shared by many who have been tested."

Genetic Testing Can Aid Those at Risk of Genetic Disease

Catherine V. Hayes

Catherine V. Hayes is the director of the Huntington's Disease Society, headquartered in New York. Hayes has a family history of Huntington's disease, which generally strikes its sufferers at mid- or later life. The physically and psychologically degenerative disease is transmitted genetically. In late 1983 scientists devised a test that can determine whether a person carries the Huntington's gene. Because of the debilitating nature of the disease, opinion is mixed on whether testing is beneficial. Some feel that patients who find out they carry the gene may become despondent or suicidal. Hayes, the author of the following viewpoint, asserts that for her, testing was the right thing to do. She believes that with the proper foundation, individuals and families can benefit from being tested.

As you read, consider the following questions:

1. Why does Hayes believe the decision to be tested for Huntington's disease should be a family decision?
2. Why does the author believe the test for Huntington's is beneficial, even for those who are told that they carry the gene for the disease?

Adapted from Catherine V. Hayes, "Genetic Testing for Huntington's Disease—A Family Issue," *The New England Journal of Medicine*, vol. 327, no. 20, November 12, 1992. (The original article contains references and graphics not reproduced here.) Reprinted with permission.

For the first 33 years of my life, I lived at risk for Huntington's disease. Huntington's disease is transmitted in an autosomal dominant fashion: each child of a person with the disease has a 50-50 chance of inheriting the Huntington's gene. Though it may take decades for symptoms to become apparent (Huntington's disease usually strikes insidiously between the ages of 30 and 50), the gene will eventually cause the disease and lead to death after 10 to 15 years of unremitting degeneration.

As a child, I discovered the well-kept family secret that my maternal grandfather had lived out his last years in a state mental hospital suffering from Huntington's disease. I watched an aunt and uncle slowly succumb to the disease. Finally, I had to admit that my mother was also affected. My brothers and I were now, unmistakably, at risk.

Before 1983, the anxious uncertainty of those of us at risk for Huntington's disease could be brought to an end either by a positive diagnosis or by the onset of old age and the increasing likelihood that we were among the lucky ones—the "escapees." We had to wait, watch for minor twitching, mood swings, and forgetfulness, and hope that they did not become severe enough to confirm our worst fears. We knew that if Huntington's disease developed there was (and still is) nothing to be done.

One fall day in 1983, I heard on the car radio that a genetic marker, a segment of DNA believed to be close to the gene for Huntington's disease, had been discovered. It was clear to me that within a few years a presymptomatic test would be available. I had to stop the car because I was crying. I knew that I would take the test. Knowing, whatever the outcome, would be better than waiting and wondering day after day.

A presymptomatic test was indeed developed in 1986, and in the summer of 1987 I enrolled in the testing research project at Johns Hopkins University Hospital. It was a long and complex process. Blood samples from numerous members of my family had to be collected and analyzed. I underwent several months of genetic counseling to clarify my motivation and to determine my ability to cope with any possible outcome. After a period of months, nothing remained but the nerve-racking wait for the results.

Finally, the wait was over: my test was negative. The DNA analysis had shown with 96 percent certainty (later increased to 99 percent, with refinement of the testing process) that I had not inherited the gene for Huntington's disease. When I learned the results I cried and laughed. It took months for the news to sink in. I am still adjusting.

Incomparable Relief

The incomparable relief I felt at finally being free of the fear and uncertainty (a feeling shared by many who have been tested) was tempered by the painful knowledge that other family members had not been and would not be so lucky. I have five brothers and eight nieces and nephews. One brother already has symptoms. He has two children. Another brother has been tested and, like me, received a negative result. He has married and had his first child. A third brother, also with two children, took the test and was found to have a high probability of having the Huntington's gene.

As president of the Huntington's Disease Society of America, I have learned that many medical professionals have difficulty viewing genetic issues in a family context. This is not surprising given the conventional emphasis in medicine on individuals. Moreover, the care of a person with a chronic and complex disorder such as Huntington's disease places a heavy demand on an overburdened health care system ill equipped to address secondary issues involving "unaffected" family members.

Nevertheless, a diagnosis of Huntington's disease affects every member of the family. Families and family members deal with it in various ways. Some people confront it openly, some will not talk about it, and others dwell only on the negative aspects. In short, no one can control how families will handle genetic issues, nor can anyone predict individual coping strategies. For example, there is often a nosy relative intent on piecing together a family pedigree (and other family members who insist on absolute privacy). I believe strongly that researchers should not feel compelled to do anything about such situations. Inquisitive relatives are a part of every family, and if the family can do nothing to quell their curiosity, then neither can anyone else.

A Family Issue

Nonetheless, some general guidelines might be useful in dealing with families. First and foremost, genetic testing must be viewed as a family issue, not an individual one. The person who enrolls in a testing program should be strongly encouraged to involve other family members, within reason. Testing one member of a family will affect other members. Persons who refuse to involve their families may not have considered fully the consequences for other members or for themselves.

A case in point involves a pair of identical twins, only one of whom wanted to be tested. She swore that she would never reveal the results to anyone else in the family, in particular her twin. The researchers agreed to test her. Once she was informed of the results—that there was a high probability that she would have Huntington's disease—the information spread quickly throughout the entire family. This meant that the twin who did not want to know her genetic status was now faced with the unwelcome knowledge that she too would probably have the disease. Had the researchers considered all the implications of testing, they might have referred both sisters for family counseling, providing them the opportunity to resolve the question of whether to be tested. One person's right to know in this case did not necessarily outweigh her twin's right not to know. When information was given to one twin, the other irretrievably lost the freedom to decide.

Huntington's Test Offers Relief

The results [of our survey] suggest that predictive testing for Huntington's disease may maintain or even improve the psychological well-being of many people at risk. As expected, most of those who received a result indicating a decreased risk showed marked improvement in psychological health, as evaluated by our three primary measures of psychological status. As compared with this group, those who received a result indicating an increased risk have not derived the same psychological benefit. However, they have not responded to predictive testing in the negative manner that was feared when programs of predictive testing for Huntington's disease were first developed. Moreover, as compared with those who received a result indicating no change in their degree of risk, both the increased-risk group and the decreased-risk group reported less depression and a greater sense of psychological well-being at the 12-month follow-up assessment. Knowing the result of the predictive test, even if it indicates an increased risk, reduces uncertainty and provides an opportunity for appropriate planning. Therefore, as our findings suggest, people who receive informative results, regardless of the content, may derive psychological benefits not experienced by those who remain uncertain.

Sandi Wiggins et al., *The New England Journal of Medicine*, November 12, 1992.

Most researchers cannot possibly know what it is like to grow up in a family haunted by a genetic disease—nor should we expect them to. But a greater effort to empathize could help improve their understanding of families and enhance the relationship between doctors and families. This point was most clearly illustrated for me during a recent symposium on genetic diseases. One participant reported that 25 percent of family members in a survey said they would terminate a pregnancy in which the baby faced a "serious medical issue," but not one in which the baby would have the same disability as the respondent. Most of the participants shook their heads in disbelief. For me and for people like me, this was no surprise. We grow up among family members affected by a genetic disorder. They are real people to us, our own flesh and blood. We are accustomed to the changes that the disease brings about, and although we may be fearful, we love and value our affected relatives. For many of us, abortion might be the best option when there is a risk of some other medical condition, but not our own.

Suicide Threat

Another difficult moral issue is that of suicide when the likelihood of having a genetic disease becomes known. It has been speculated that genetic testing may lead to an increased rate of suicide among those who test positive. To date, post-testing follow-up has not borne out this hypothesis. The possibility of suicide is greater when symptoms begin to appear than in the immediate aftermath of testing. Obviously, the topic of suicide should be carefully probed in the early stages of genetic counseling. When it is discussed, counselors will generally find that they are not exploring virgin territory. Most people at risk for Huntington's disease have thought long and hard about what they might do if symptoms develop and may even admit these thoughts. Most of those who actually ask for genetic information are relatively prepared to handle the facts.

The rapidly advancing field of molecular genetics will eventually have far-reaching consequences for everyone. Although Huntington's disease continues to be a closely guarded secret in some families, for others radical changes in science are already being matched by radical changes in attitude. There are clear signs of an emergent openness about the disease. My grandfather lived out his last days in an institution, and I did not even know he was alive. My five brothers married and most had children before we openly acknowledged the existence of Huntington's disease in our family. But my 15-year-old nephew has readily stood up in class and told his fellow students about Huntington's disease (in contrast to his teacher, who in reviewing various conditions had difficulty pronouncing "Huntington's disease"). My older brother (who has Huntington's disease) recently agreed to be featured in *People* magazine.

Of course, denial still exists. My mother, who has lived in a nursing home for years now, still tells me that she does not have "that disease." Denial is after all a valuable coping mechanism, particularly for people who have little else to fall back on. It should not be taken away until there is something better—effective treatment, a cure—to replace it. Many people who said they would be tested have changed their minds. This is understandable to those of us at risk for Huntington's disease. In the abstract, it is easy to think that you would want to know. When it is time to find out, the possibility of a positive test is frightening. How many of us would really choose to be told how we will die?

285

Perhaps I sound as if I am opposed to genetic testing. I am not—I took the test myself—but I do believe the test should be approached by all parties with the utmost caution and that it should not be undertaken without safeguards. I am simply a proponent of what one genetic counselor calls "devil's advocate counseling." The Huntington's Disease Society of America has incorporated this approach into its own predictive-testing guidelines. Prospective participants are encouraged to attend numerous counseling sessions to explore fully their motivation for taking the test and their likely reactions to any possible outcome. They are urged to bring a friend with them when the results are reported. They are then encouraged to return for follow-up counseling sessions. Some consider this approach to be overkill. As genetic testing becomes more and more widespread, the counseling component will become increasingly difficult to enforce. And once the gene for Huntington's disease is isolated, the process will probably be reduced to a simple blood test. But for now, as we continue to learn about the real-life consequences of revealing potentially explosive genetic information, these guidelines or safeguards are probably necessary, not only for persons at risk who wish to be tested, but also for those doing the testing.

Yet, however carefully we tread, we will always be picking our way through a minefield. It is impossible to know what effect the predictive test for Huntington's disease will have on anyone—the affected parent, who passed on the gene, the children, who might inherit the gene, other relatives, employers, or friends. It is encouraging, but not surprising, that [the study on the psychological consequences of testing for Huntington's disease conducted by S. Wiggins et al.] found that just getting an answer—any answer—increased one's sense of well-being by removing the uncertainty. We are all different, but for most of us an answer helps by eliminating the daily worrying and by allowing time for planning. It is by working together that we can provide more answers to those who want them. I urge more open communication among medical professionals, families—who have a great deal to offer in the way of experience—and volunteer organizations, which can serve as a bridge between the other two groups.

"If you have any type of hereditary illness, you can pretty much forget about insurance coverage."

Genetic Testing Will Lead to Discrimination

Theresa Morelli, interviewed by Vicki Quade

Attorney Theresa Morelli's father was diagnosed as having Huntington's disease, a debilitating and degenerative chorea, transmitted genetically, that usually develops in adult life and progresses to dementia. Although Morelli herself had no symptoms of Huntington's, her father's medical records prevented her from obtaining health insurance. Morelli now advocates for privacy of genetic information. In the following viewpoint, an interview with Morelli for the American Bar Association's *Human Rights* magazine, Morelli expresses the fear held by many that genetic testing will lead to widespread economic discrimination by employers and insurance companies. Vicki Quade, who interviewed Morelli, is editor of *Human Rights*.

As you read, consider the following questions:

1. According to the author, why would insurance carriers be likely to discriminate against those known to carry genes for such diseases as Huntington's?
2. Why does Morelli think insurance companies are not justified in denying coverage based on genetic information? Do you agree with her? Explain.

Theresa Morelli was denied insurance coverage when the under-writer learned that her father was diagnosed with Huntington's disease, a progressive neurological disorder. She was 29 at the time, in good health, and furious. The insurance company did not offer to exclude coverage for HD or offer her coverage at a higher premium.

She eventually got disability coverage under a group policy through the American Trial Lawyers Association. She also later learned that her father's diagnosis was incorrect—his physicians now believe he has a progressive form of Alzheimer's.

Without legislative protection, she believes, families affected by genetic disorders and genetic predispositions will be uninsurable and forced onto the welfare and Medicaid rolls. She is now a lawyer with a mission—to secure federal legislation protecting the privacy of genetic information from insurers, banks, schools, and other institutions. "We must prevent this abuse of biotechnology before it's too late," she says. . . .

This interview, recorded in Morelli's office, was conducted by Human Rights *editor Vicki Quade.*

HR: Who has the right to genetic information and how should it be used?

TM: The health care provider has a right to that information, but there must be voluntary consent by the test taker and confidentiality to ensure that the information isn't misused by an insurance company, employer, or another health care provider.

HR: Explain how insurance companies use family medical histories and the results of genetic testing.

TM: Insurance companies look at family histories, and if a family member has a genetic disorder, especially if it's a parent, they're going to deny coverage.

Now, they won't tell you this.

I've asked the Health Insurance Association of America [HIAA] and the American Council of Life Insurance [ACLI] to give me a copy of their underwriting manuals, and they still haven't. I actually got those manuals from another source.

If you have any type of hereditary illness, you can pretty much forget about insurance coverage.

I'm now hearing about people with genetic predispositions not being able to get insurance or workers' compensation. The most egregious case I saw was two years ago. A guy came in with what he thought was a malpractice case. As I looked at the case, I said, "You don't have malpractice here, but let me see what your workers' compensation records say."

He couldn't get workers' compensation because he has genetic arteriosclerosis. The company denied him after he gave them his family medical history. So now his union is fighting for him. It could take two or three years for the union to get him workers' comp.

HR: How do insurance companies get this information?

TM: It's given by providers. Sometimes it's given by the individual.

In my situation, I applied for disability income protection. I paid my premium up front. I had a medical exam. And then I signed a release for my records.

My whole family had the same doctor. My father's diagnosis of Huntington's disease was written on the front of my file, so when the office sent a copy of my file to the insurance company, my father's diagnosis was right there.

Providers give information away all the time. If it's not written in your file, it's there under a diagnostic code.

When it's genetic, they've got to be careful because insurance companies will red flag anything hereditary or genetic in origin.

"Private" Information

HR: Isn't any of that information private?

TM: It's supposed to be private.

In my situation, the doctor's office had no right to give my father's diagnosis, but they did it inadvertently.

You know, whenever you apply for life or disability insurance, the information you provide is registered with the Medical Information Bureau in Boston, a national centralized data bank. They claim that health care information isn't sent there, but I'm not really sure of that.

For the rest of your life, that information is there and any insurance company can tap into that.

You can have your file purged. You have to write MIB and ask to see your file. I've never seen one actually come back. Usually they say they don't have anything on you.

Say you're lucky enough that they send you a file. If you want something erroneous or detrimental deleted, they mark your file "delete."

So when you apply for insurance and insurance companies see the word "delete," it's a red flag to them.

It seems like you can't get away from this. If the erroneous or bad information is there, it's bad. But if they see "delete," they'll put two and two together.

HR: How widespread is the discrimination being practiced by insurance companies?

TM: Insurance companies contend that it doesn't exist.

Dr. Paul Billings at Pacific Presbyterian Hospital in San Francisco, who is the premier genetic-bias researcher, has documented at least 50 cases.

Currently Dr. Billings is undertaking a bigger study. He has written to 1,000 people and he told me he's already gotten back 870 responses. Now he'll spend time verifying every episode of discrimination.

The National Society of Genetic Counselors is also tabulating this. During testimony before Congress about the misuse of genetic information, they presented at least 20 cases of discrimination.

It's widespread, but insurance companies will have you believe it's nonexistent.

Insurance Not for All

Insurers' arguments defending the need to classify risk (and, thereby, to screen for genetic conditions), are founded in the notion that risk classification makes good business sense. Insurers readily admit that such a system leaves certain people uninsurable, but do not believe that they should be held responsible for that problem. It is not the intent of the insurance industry to ensure access to health care for all, nor does the industry perceive its responsibility to be one of facilitating equality of outcome. . . .

If the laws and regulations governing the practice of insurance in this country do not change, the genetic testing that will be made possible as we continue to map the human genome may result in many more individuals being denied private insurance coverage than ever before.

Nancy E. Kass, *Hastings Center Report*, November/December 1992.

HR: Are insurance companies concerned about genetic diseases because they've been burdened by the AIDS crisis? Is it that they don't want another major drain on their resources?

TM: They claim people are going to buy up all kinds of policies. And then when they get the disease, either they'll leave a rich family or they'll have all kinds of disability income rolling in.

I've talked with a lot of people about this and only one very distraught individual even said a thing like that to me. Most people just want one policy so they can help their families.

Insurance companies don't even give people the chance to ask for higher premiums. They don't give you a chance to say, "Well, exclude the hereditary illness. Let me have insurance for everything else." At this point it's all or nothing.

There have also been documented discrimination cases involving fetuses that were found to have genetic defects.

One was a cystic fibrosis case. One was adult-onset polycystic kidney disease. The HMO [Health Maintenance Organization] said, "If you carry the fetus to term, we will not pay the child's medical expenses or for your pregnancy."

What is that telling the parents? That's telling them that if you don't abort the fetus, you're going to be stuck with its care for the rest of your life.

I told this to one of the senior counsel at ACLI, who said to me, "Well, if that happened, you just sue the insurance company." I said to her, "You have an expectant couple on your hands—who can afford to wait three or four years for a lawsuit until you know?"

That's their response. If your insurance company forces you to have an abortion, you just sue the insurance company. Or have your baby, then sue. . . .

Impact of Genetic Information

Looking into the future, we have to start considering the impact of genetic information that will be available at birth. Say you have something like Huntington's in your family. Can you be denied admission to graduate school? Would it be harder to get into law school, medical school? Will you be able to get a loan?

Could someone say, "You can't have a mortgage because you're a terrible risk"? Could someone say, "I'm sorry, you can't adopt because you have a hereditary illness and might not be able to care for this child"?

HR: Why shouldn't insurance companies have access to genetic information?

TM: One major reason is interpretation.

About 4,000 genetic diseases have already been identified. But a statistic by itself isn't going to tell you when you're going to get the disease or the severity of it. It just tells you that you have a predisposition.

I asked HIAA, "How do your underwriters deal with genetic diseases? Do you have doctors there? Do you have nurses?" And I was told, "We don't have enough money to have what you're talking about."

Which means people with four-year degrees in business are making these decisions. And they tell me for the more hairy situations they'll send it to a nurse or somebody to review.

There have to be controls on how the information is used, and until those controls exist, we have to limit who has access to the information.

HR: Could genetic testing ever be required in the future?

TM: Wisconsin is the only state I know of that has outlawed it.

It's not illegal at this point for insurance companies in all other states to require genetic testing.

HR: Do you envision a new genetic elitism, or racism, developing?

TM: Yes I do, especially if you look at how HMOs are already practicing genetic elitism by telling parents they won't cover the medical care of a fetus with a genetic disease.

The area that bothers me most is gene manipulation. I'm veering off a bit, but this shows the danger of misuse when you're talking about genetic possibilities.

There are two types of gene therapy.

In one type, you treat a body cell because it's diseased. If you have a sick kid, you can sometimes tinker with the genes so that child gets better.

Then you have a different kind of gene manipulation that's in the experimentation stage right now. You can tinker with the genes of an unborn child, change its obesity, sexual orientation, height, intelligence. Change it for all other generations.

The Lou Harris people were commissioned by the March of Dimes to do a poll. The shocking results showed that 68 percent of respondents didn't know anything about gene therapy or genetic testing. But 42 percent were all in favor of gene manipulation to change their child's obesity. And I think 33 percent said that they would tinker with intelligence genes of their child. This is not to cure a child. Just to make it better.

And I fear that if this becomes available on a wide scale, you'll see a lot of wealthy white people doing this for their children. If we're not careful we could be looking at another eugenics age.

We're trying to get Congress to see the potential here of hurting minorities and women.

HR: You've argued that the information gleaned from the Human Genome Project will be ripe for abuse. How could it be used against the public?

TM: At this time, only 12 or 13 classical genetic tests have been developed. These are tests for muscular dystrophy, cystic fibrosis, other classic genetic diseases. As more tests are developed, there will just be more information available for the insurance industry to use against people.

It's been predicted by the top biological and clinical geneticists that in a matter of 10 years we'll have a simple blood test that will give a genetic profile of newborns.

So once they have a genetic profile on you, how's that information going to be used? Insurance companies are going to love that.

Periodical Bibliography

The following articles have been selected to supplement the diverse views presented in this chapter.

Anna Aldovini and Richard A. Young	"The New Vaccines," *Technology Review*, January 1992.
American Journal of Law & Medicine	Special issue on "The Human Genome Initiative and the Impact of Genetic Testing and Screening Technologies," vol. 17, nos. 1 & 2, 1991. Available from 765 Commonwealth Ave., Boston, MA 02215.
Judy Berlfein	"The Earliest Warning," *Discover*, February 1992.
Paul Billings	"Screened Out," *Christian Social Action*, January 1991.
Council for Responsible Genetics	Position papers on genetic discrimination and the Human Genome Initiative, *Issues in Reproductive and Genetic Engineering*, vol. 3, no. 3, 1990. Available from Pergamon Press, 660 White Plains Rd., Tarrytown, NY 10591.
Council on Ethical and Judicial Affairs, American Medical Association	"Use of Genetic Testing by Employers," *JAMA*, October 2, 1991.
Elaine Draper	"Genetic Secrets: Social Issues of Medical Screening in a Genetic Age," *Hastings Center Report*, July/August 1992.
Sharon J. Durfy and Amy E. Grotevant	"The Human Genome Project," *Kennedy Institute of Ethics Journal*, December 1991. Available from Georgetown University, Washington, DC 20057.
Troy Duster	"Assessing the Quality of Life," *Christian Social Action*, January 1991.
Rochelle Green	"Tinkering with the Secrets of Life," *Health*, January 1990.
Gayle Hanson	"At a Price: Exploring the Mystery of Genes," *Insight*, December 28, 1992. Available from PO Box 91022, Washington, D.C. 20090-1022.
Richard Hatchett	"Brave New Worlds: Perspective on the American Experience of Eugenics," *The Pharos*, Fall 1991.

Journal of Clinical Ethics	Special section on genetic testing for Huntington's disease and "The Ethical Use of Technology in Genetics," Winter 1991. Available from 107 E. Church St., Frederick, MD 21701.
Elizabeth Kristol	"Picture Perfect: The Politics of Prenatal Testing," *First Things*, April 1993. Available from 156 Fifth Ave., Ste. 400, New York, NY 10010.
Abby Lippman	"Mother Matters: A Fresh Look at Prenatal Genetic Testing," *Issues in Reproductive and Genetic Engineering*, vol. 5, no. 2, 1992.
Thomas H. Murray	"Genetics and the Moral Mission of Health Insurance," *Hastings Center Report*, November/December 1992.
The New Internationalist	March 1991. Whole issue devoted to biotechnology.
David Orentlicher	"Genetic Screening by Employers," *JAMA*, February 16, 1990.
Stephen G. Post	"Euthanasia and Prenatal Genetic Testin," *The World & I*, March 1993.
Andrew Purvis	"Laying Siege to a Deadly Gene," *Time*, February 24, 1992.
Leslie Roberts	"To Test or Not to Test?" *Science*, January 5, 1990.
Harmon L. Smith	"Genetic Technologies: Can We Do Responsibly Everything We Can Do Technically?" *National Forum*, Winter 1992. Available from PO Box 16000, Louisiana State University, Baton Rouge, LA 70893.
Anne Waldschmidt	*Issues in Reproductive and Genetic Engineering*, vol. 5, no. 2, 1992.
Darrell E. Ward	"Gene Therapy: The Splice of Life," *USA Today*, January 1993.
Robert A. Weinberg	"The Dark Side of the Genome," *Technology Review*, April 1991.
Wilson Quarterly	Spring 1992. Several articles devoted to advances in genetic engineering.
Robert Wright	"Achilles' Helix," *The New Republic*, July 9 & 16, 1990.

For Further Discussion

Chapter 1

1. Do you think human by-products should be allowed to be patented as an incentive to continuing research? Do you think that scientific research would "dry up" if patents were not allowed on research products? Explain.

2. Do you think George J. Annas would approve of the three-tier classification system devised by Margaret S. Swain and Randy W. Marusyk for determining patentability? Explain.

3. Which viewpoint on human experimentation do you find more convincing? Why? List three facts from that viewpoint that helped persuade you.

Chapter 2

1. In general, what do you think of the advances made in organ transplantation? Do you think that, overall, such advances are beneficial or detrimental to humankind? Explain.

2. Do you agree with authors Kass, Fox, and Swazey that organ transplantation raises issues of dehumanization? Explain.

3. Do you think buying and selling organs is a good or bad idea? Explain.

Chapter 3

1. Do you believe the use of electively aborted fetal tissue should be allowed in research and medical treatment? What facts influence your answer? What values influence your answer?

2. Many scientists believe that the 1988 moratorium on federal funding of fetal tissue research severely hampered an important area of biomedical research. Others say the moratorium allowed emphasis to be placed on alternative methods of treating disease that might not otherwise have been developed. What do you think about the government's refusing to fund research on the basis of moral conviction?

3. Some people compare fetal tissue research to the research Nazi scientists performed on living people during World War II. What do you think of this comparison? Explain your answer.

4. If one of your loved ones could be saved from a debilitating or fatal disease by the use of aborted fetal tissue, would you accept that treatment? What if the needed tissue was to come from a sick elderly person who would die as a result of the tissue removal? Do you think the situations are comparable? Explain.

Chapter 4

1. Based on the readings in this chapter, do you think that the new reproductive technologies are mostly beneficial or mostly harmful? Explain.

2. List three facts and three opinions from the viewpoints that favor the new reproductive technologies and that you find particularly persuasive. List three facts and three opinions that are critical of the new reproductive technologies and that you find particularly persuasive.

3. Recent court cases relating to surrogate motherhood have issued conflicting rulings on the status of the gestational mother (the one who bears the child) and the nurturant mother (the one who raises the child). The gestational mother has been called a womb for rent, the biological mother, and the actual mother. The nurturant mother has been called the biological mother (when her egg was used in the surrogacy process), the adoptive mother, and the actual mother. How would you define the roles of the two women? Why?

4. Some feminists laud the new reproductive technologies as allowing women greater freedom of reproductive choice than ever before. Other feminists decry these technologies as turning women into commodities and, through social pressure, actually giving them less freedom to make the choice not to have children. What is your opinion? Why?

Chapter 5

1. Do you think animals should be used in biomedical research? If so, what limitations, if any, would you place on such research?

2. *BioScience* magazine recently stated that "creative research [using animals and] having no immediate medical benefit is both proper and necessary, because it is the foundation on which science builds." Do you agree with this statement? Explain your opinion.

3. Those who defend animal research often point to the significant advances that have been made because of it—the development of insulin, surgical techniques, anesthesia, and heart transplants, for example. Take the role of the critic of animal research: What would you say to this justification for animal research?

4. Roger E. Ulrich's viewpoint specifically talks about inadequate justification for using animals in psychological research. Which of Ulrich's arguments would apply as well to medical research? Which would not?

5. At present, most drugs and medical techniques must go through a multistep experimental process before they are approved by the government for general use on human patients. The last two steps include use on animals and limited use on humans. Based on the readings in this chapter, do you think either the animal or the human part of the process could safely be eliminated? Which viewpoint most strongly influences your opinion? Explain.

6. Compare the two viewpoints about organ transplants from animals to humans: Which uses more facts? Which uses more opinions? Which do you find more persuasive? Why?

Chapter 6

1. Genetic engineering offers the promise of ridding human life of much hereditary disease. It also offers the possibility of increasing discrimination against those who are different. Based on the readings in this chapter, do you think genetic research should continue to be funded by the government? Explain.

2. Do you think insurance companies and employers should be able to obtain the results of genetic tests? Why or why not? Take the role of an insurance company executive. How would you answer this question? Take the role of a person with Huntington's disease in your family history. How would you answer this question?

3. List three facts found in viewpoints in this chapter that you find convincing support for genetic research. List three facts that you find convincing against genetic research. Which side do you find stronger? Explain.

Organizations to Contact

The editors have compiled the following list of organizations that are concerned with the issues debated in this book. All have publications or information available for interested readers. For best results, allow as much time as possible for the organizations to respond. The descriptions below are derived from materials provided by the organizations. This list was compiled upon the date of publication. Names, addresses, and phone numbers of organizations are subject to change.

American Anti-Vivisection Society
Suite 204 Nobel Plaza
801 Old York Rd.
Jenkintown, PA 19046-1685
(215) 887-0816

The oldest animal rights group in America, the society opposes all animal experimentation. It publishes educational pamphlets and the monthly *AV* magazine.

American Association for Laboratory Animal Science (AALAS)
70 Timber Creek, Suite 5
Cordova, TN 38018
(901) 754-8620

AALAS is concerned with the production, use, care, and study of animals used in biomedical research. It serves as a clearinghouse for information on the procurement, care, and management of laboratory animals. The association publishes two bimonthlies, the newsletter *AALAS Bulletin* and the journal *Laboratory Animal Science*.

American Association of Tissue Banks
1350 Beverly Rd., Suite 220-A
McLean, VA 22101
(703) 827-9582

The association's goals are to encourage the development of regional tissue banks and to establish guidelines and standards for the harvesting, preservation, distribution, and use of tissues for transplantation. Its publications include technical manuals and the book *Standards for Tissue Banking and Surgical Bone Banking*.

American Fertility Society
2140 Eleventh Ave. S., Suite 200
Birmingham, AL 35205-2800
(205) 987-5000

The society is made up of physicians, veterinarians, researchers, and others concerned about the reproductive health of humans and animals. It seeks to extend knowledge of all aspects of fertility and problems of infertility and reproduction. This is accomplished by offering client services, conducting workshops, and providing a forum for reproductive studies. Publications of the society include the quarterly newsletter *Fertility News* and the monthly journal *Fertility and Sterility*.

American Fund for Alternatives to Animal Research
c/o Dr. Ethel Thurston
175 W. Twelfth St., No. 16-G
New York, NY 10011
(212) 989-8073

The fund sponsors research that does not use animals. It seeks to show that many animal experiments are unnecessary and to save laboratory animals from painful tests. It also lobbies the government to subsidize more research to find alternatives to animal experimentation. In addition to pamphlets, press releases, and action alerts, the fund publishes *International Animal Action* semiannually and *Affair News Abstracts* three times a year.

American Medical Association (AMA)
515 N. State St.
Chicago, IL 60610
(312) 464-5000

The AMA is the largest and most prestigious professional association for medical doctors. It helps set standards for medical education and practices and is a powerful lobby in Washington for physicians' interests. The association publishes monthly journals for many medical fields, including the *Archives of Pathology and Laboratory Medicine* and the *Archives of Surgery*, as well as the weekly *Journal of the American Medical Association*.

Association of Biotechnology Companies (ABC)
1666 Connecticut Ave. NW, Suite 330
Washington, DC 20009-1039
(202) 234-3330

ABC provides information to its members on biotechnology issues pertaining to regulations, patents, and finances. Its publications include the bimonthly newsletter *American Biotechnology Companies* and the periodic *ABC Alerts*.

Beauty Without Cruelty, USA
175 W. Twelfth St., No. 16-G
New York, NY 10011
(212) 989-8073

Beauty Without Cruelty opposes the use of animals in laboratory testing done to develop cosmetics and the killing of animals for their fur. It works to educate the public about the suffering of animals in laboratories, fur farms, and wildlife trapping enterprises. The organization provides information on cruelty-free products and simulated fur fashions and where to purchase them. It publishes the *Compassionate Shopper* newsletter three times a year, as well as leaflets and the triannual *Action Alert*.

Center for Biomedical Ethics
Box 33 UMHC
Minneapolis, MN 55455
(612) 625-4917

The center seeks to advance and disseminate knowledge concerning ethical issues in health care and the life sciences. It conducts original research, offers educational programs, fosters public discussion and debate, and assists in the formulation of public policy. The center publishes a quarterly newsletter and reading packets on specific topics, including organ transplants and fetal tissue research.

Center for Surrogate Parenting
8383 Wilshire Blvd., Suite 750
Beverly Hills, CA 90211
(213) 655-1974

The center works to disseminate current and accurate information on the legal, moral, ethical, and psychological aspects of surrogate parenting and establishes ethical and procedural guidelines for new laws protecting those involved in surrogate parenting. It publishes a semiannual newsletter, *Center for Surrogate Parenting*, as well as information sheets and brochures.

Council for Responsible Genetics
186 South St., 4th Fl.
Boston, MA 02111
(617) 868-0870

The council counts among its members scientists, medical professionals, trade unionists, feminists, and peace activists. It monitors and analyzes the biotechnology industry and discusses the social implications of new biotechnology developments. A bimonthly newsletter published by the council is titled *GeneWatch*.

Fertility Research Foundation
1430 Second Ave., Suite 103
New York, NY 10021
(212) 744-5500

The foundation conducts research on numerous aspects of human reproduction and provides therapeutic, diagnostic, and consultative services for childless couples. It publishes the quarterly *Infertility Journal*.

Foundation for Biomedical Research
818 Connecticut Ave. NW
Washington, DC 20006
(202) 457-0654

The foundation supports humane animal research and serves to inform and educate the public about the necessity and importance of laboratory animals in biomedical research and testing. It publishes a bimonthly newsletter, videos and films, and numerous background papers, including *The Use of Animals in Biomedical Research and Testing* and *Caring for Laboratory Animals*.

Hastings Center
255 Elm Rd.
Briarcliff Manor, NY 10510
(914) 762-8500

Since its founding in 1969, the center has played a central role in responding to advances in medicine, the biological sciences, and the social sciences by raising ethical questions related to such advances. It conducts research on ethical issues and provides consultations. The center publishes books, papers, guidelines, and the bimonthly *Hastings Center Report*.

Incurably Ill for Animal Research
PO Box 1873
Bridgeview, IL 60455
(708) 598-7787

The organization consists of people who have incurable diseases and who are concerned that the use of animals in medical research will be stopped or severely limited by animal rights activists, thus delaying or preventing the discovery or development of new cures. It publishes a monthly *Bulletin* and a quarterly *Newsletter*.

Living Bank
PO Box 6725
Houston, TX 77265
(713) 528-2971

The bank is a national registry and referral service created to help those persons who, upon death, wish to donate organs and/or tissue for transplantation, therapy, or research. It provides educational materials on organ donation and publishes a quarterly newsletter, *Bank Account*.

National Association for Biomedical Research (NABR)
818 Connecticut Ave. NW, Suite 303
Washington, DC 20006
(202) 857-0540

NABR is an organization comprising universities, research institutes, professional societies, animal breeders and suppliers, and pharmaceutical companies that use animals for biomedical research and testing. NABR also monitors and, if necessary, attempts to influence government legislation regarding the use of animals in research and testing. Its publications include the biweekly *NABR Update* and the *NABR Alert*, published six to ten times a year.

People for the Ethical Treatment of Animals (PETA)
Box 42516
Washington, DC 20015
(301) 770-7444

PETA is an educational and activist group that opposes all forms of animal exploitation. It conducts rallies and demonstrations to focus attention on animal experimentation, the fur fashion industry, and the killing of animals for human consumption—three issues it considers institutionalized cruelty. Through the use of films, slides, and pictures, PETA hopes to educate the public about human chauvinist attitudes toward animals and about the conditions in slaughterhouses and research laboratories. It publishes reports on animal experimentation and animal farming and periodic *People for the Ethical Treatment of Animals—Action Alerts*.

Transplantation Society
c/o Ronald W. Ferguson, M.D.
Ohio State University
Dept. of Surgery
Means Hall, Rm. 258
1654 Ugham Dr.
Columbus, OH 43210
(614) 293-8545

The society is composed of physicians and scientists who have made significant contributions to the advancement of knowledge in transplantation biology and medicine. The purpose of the society is to increase and promote information about transplantation. It publishes *Transplantation* monthly and *Transplantation Proceedings* quarterly.

United Network for Organ Sharing (UNOS)
1100 Boulders Pkwy., Suite 500
Richmond, VA 23225
(804) 330-8500

UNOS is a system of transplant and organ procurement centers, tissue-typing labs, and transplant surgical teams. It was formed to help organ donors and people who need organs to find each other. By law, organs used for transplants must be cleared through UNOS. The network also formulates and implements national policies on equal access to organs and organ allocation, organ procurement, and AIDS testing. It publishes the monthly *UNOS Update*.

Bibliography of Books

Kenneth D. Alprin, ed.	*The Ethics of Reproductive Technology.* New York: Oxford University Press, 1992.
Robert M. Baird and Stuart E. Rosenbaum, eds.	*Animal Experimentation: The Moral Issues.* Buffalo: Prometheus Books, 1991.
Diane M. Bartels et al., eds.	*Beyond Baby M: Ethical Issues in New Reproductive Techniques.* Totowa, NJ: Humana Press, 1990.
Jerry E. Bishop and Michael Waldholz	*Genome: The Story of the Most Astonishing Scientific Adventure of Our Time . . . .* New York: Simon & Schuster 1990.
Robert H. Blank	*Regulating Reproduction.* New York: Columbia University Press, 1990.
Robert H. Blank and Andrea L. Bonnickson, eds.	*Emerging Issues in Biomedical Policy: An Annual Review.* Vol. 2. New York: Columbia University Press, 1993.
Ruth Ellen Bulger, Elizabeth Heitman, and Stanley Joel Rieser, eds.	*The Ethical Dimensions of the Biological Sciences.* New York: Cambridge University Press, 1993.
Arthur L. Caplan	*If I Were a Rich Man Could I Buy a Pancreas? and Other Essays on the Ethics of Health Care.* Bloomington: Indiana University Press, 1992.
Arthur L. Caplan, ed.	*When Medicine Went Bad: Bioethics and the Holocaust.* Totowa, NJ: Humana Press, 1992.
Arthur L. Caplan and Dorothy Vawter	*The Use of Human Fetal Tissue: Scientific, Ethical, and Policy Concerns.* Minneapolis: University of Minnesota Press, 1990.
Russ Carman	*The Illusions of Animal Rights.* Iola, WI: Krause Publications, 1990.
Bernard D. Davis, ed.	*The Genetic Revolution: Scientific Prospects and Public Perceptions.* Baltimore: Johns Hopkins University Press, 1991.
Elaine Draper	*Risky Business: Genetic Testing and Exclusionary Practices in the Hazardous Workplace.* New York: Cambridge University Press, 1991.
Troy Duster	*Backdoor to Eugenics.* New York: Routledge, 1990.
Debra Evans	*Without Moral Limits: Women, Reproduction, and the New Medical Technology.* Westchester, IL: Crossway Books, 1990.

Claire Feinman, ed.	*The Criminalization of a Woman's Body*. New York: Harrington Park Press, 1992.
Harley E. Flack and Edmund D. Pellegrino, eds.	*African-American Perspectives on Biomedical Ethics*. Washington, DC: Georgetown University Press, 1992.
Michael W. Fox	*Inhumane Society*. New York: St. Martin's Press, 1990.
Warren Freedman	*Legal Issues in Biotechnology and Human Reproduction: Artificial Conception and Modern Genetics*. New York: Quorum Books, 1991.
Marlene Gerber Fried	*From Abortion to Reproductive Freedom*. Boston: South End Press, 1990.
Larry Gostin, ed.	*Surrogate Motherhood: Politics and Privacy*. Bloomington: Indiana University Press, 1990.
John Harris	*Wonderwoman and Superman: The Ethics of Human Biotechnology*. New York: Oxford University Press, 1992.
Pat Stave Helmberger	*Transplants: Unwrapping the Second Gift of Life*. Minneapolis: Chronimed Publishing, 1992.
David Heyd	*Genethics: Moral Issues in the Creation of People*. Berkeley: University of California Press, 1992.
Robert Lee Hotz	*Designs on Life: Exploring the New Frontiers of Human Fertility*. New York: Pocket Books, 1991.
Richard T. Hull	*Ethical Issues in the New Reproductive Technologies*. Belmont, CA: Wadsworth, 1990.
James M. Humber and Robert F. Almeder, eds.	*Bioethics and the Fetus: Medical, Moral, and Legal Issues*. Totowa, NJ: Humana Press, 1991.
James M. Jasper and Dorothy Nelkin	*The Animal Rights Crusade: The Growth of a Moral Protest*. New York: Free Press, 1992.
Daniel J. Kevles and Leroy Hood, eds.	*The Code of Codes: Scientific and Social Issues in the Human Genome Project*. Cambridge, MA: Harvard University Press, 1992.
C. Don Keys and Walter Wiest, eds.	*New Harvest: Transplanting Body Parts and Reaping the Benefits*. Totowa, NJ: Humana Press, 1991.
Marque-Luisa Miringoff	*The Social Costs of Genetic Welfare*. New Brunswick, NJ: Rutgers University Press, 1991.
Benjamin A. Pierce	*The Family Genetic Sourcebook*. New York: John Wiley & Sons, 1990.
Judith Reitman	*Stolen for Profit: How the Medical Establishment Is Funding a National Pet Theft Conspiracy*. New York: Pharos Books, 1992.

Robyn Rowland   *Living Laboratories: Women and Reproductive Technologies*. Bloomington: Indiana University Press, 1992.

Kenneth E. Schemmer   *Tinkering with People*. Wheaton, IL: Victor Books, 1992.

Robert Shapiro   *The Human Blueprint: The Race to Unlock the Secret of Our Genetic Code*. New York: St. Martin's Press, 1991.

Peter Singer   *Embryo Experimentation*. New York: Cambridge University Press, 1990.

Pat Spallone   *Generation Games: Genetic Engineering and the Future for Our Lives*. London: The Women's Press, 1992.

Marilyn Strathern   *Reproducing the Future: Essays on Anthropology, Kinship, and the New Reproductive Technology*. New York: Routledge, 1992.

Elaine Sutherland
and Alexander
McCall Smith   *Family Rights: Family Law and Medical Advances*. New York: Edinburgh University Press, 1990; distributed by Columbia University Press.

Allen Verhey and
Stephen E. Lammers,
eds.   *Theological Voices in Medical Ethics*. Grand Rapids, MI: Wm. B. Eerdmans Publishing Co., 1993.

Bruce L. Wilder   *Defining the Legal Parent-Child Relationship in Alternative Reproductive Technology*. Chicago: American Bar Association, 1991.

Christopher Wills   *Exons, Introns, and Talking Genes: The Science Behind the Human Genome Project*. New York: Basic Books, 1991.

Lois Wingerson   *Mapping Our Genes: The Genome Project and the Future of Medicine*. New York: Dutton, 1990.

Steven C. Witt   *Biotechnology, Microbes, and the Environment*. San Francisco: Center for Science Information BriefBook, 1990.

Susan Wymelenberg   *Science and Babies: Private Decisions, Public Dilemmas*. Washington, DC: National Academy Press/Institute of Medicine, 1990.

Index

307

308

309

311

312